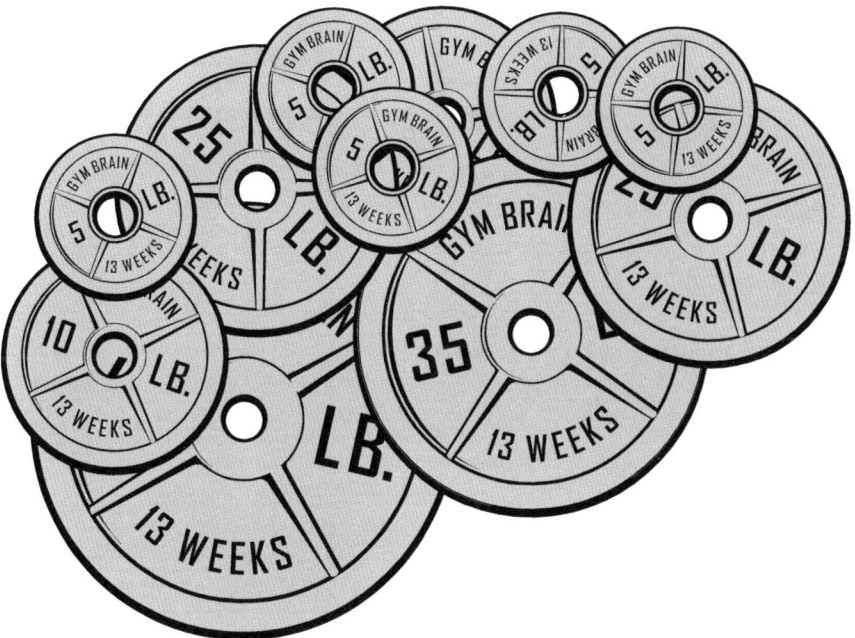

MY GYM BRAIN

A COMPREHENSIVE 13-WEEK FITNESS JOURNAL

My Gym Brain by Rachel Flint
Copyright © 2015 by Fit Like Flint, LLC
2016-2017 Edition

No part of this book may be reproduced in any form or by any means - electronic or mechanical - including photocopying, recording, or by any information storage and retrieval system without permission of the author.

All rights reserved.

Requests for information may be sent to:
Fit Like Flint, LLC
PO Box 10454
Midwest City, OK 73140
www.fitlikeflint.com

Designed by Walkingstick Design LLC, www.walkingstickdesign.com

Printed and assembled in the USA.

Scripture quotations are from The Holy Bible, English Standard Version® (ESV®), copyright © 2001 by Crossway, a publishing ministry of Good News Publishers. Used by permission. All rights reserved.

— THIS —
MY GYM BRAIN
BELONGS TO:

_____

– INTRO –

Hi! I'm Rachel Flint, creator of the MY GYM BRAIN fitness journal. As a traditionalist who loves to record workouts with pen and paper, I found that all too often, fitness journals weren't meeting my needs. There wasn't enough space to record all facets of my workouts, so I had to record extra notes in the margins. With new meal-tracking apps, I also thought the space to record meals seemed unnecessary. With so much of fitness being mental, I also wanted space to record thoughts, goals, and other notes.

I started asking fellow athletes and fitness enthusiasts what they wanted in a fitness journal. I got input from hundreds of people to make sure it would meet their needs. It had to be something useful for even the most seasoned athletes but also a valuable tool for a beginner.

Creating this journal has been a labor of love, and I'm very proud of the finished product. I'm so thankful for all the folks who gave me valuable input, and I'm excited to hear *your* feedback! If you think of a way we can make it even better, I invite you to email me directly at rachel@fitlikeflint.com. In the meantime, I hope MY GYM BRAIN serves you well and becomes your favorite way to log workouts and pursue your fitness goals.

Blessings,

Rachel

Rachel Flint is the founder and CEO of Fit Like Flint, a fitness apparel and accessory company. She is also a sponsored athlete and officer in the Air National Guard. She is married and has three children. She has won multiple transformation challenges and is dedicated to helping others reach their potential. Rachel encourages thousands through her social media accounts and private fitness groups, and now through the My Gym Brain fitness journal.

GOAL SETTING

A GOAL WELL SET IS HALF MET.
— Rachel Flint

Set S.M.A.R.T. goals!
Specific | Measurable | Attainable | Realistic | Time-Bound

"YOU GOTTA HAVE A GOAL. DO YOU HAVE A GOAL?"
-Kit, *Pretty Woman*

Set three to five S.M.A.R.T. goals for the next 13 weeks.

_____
_____
_____
_____
_____

Now that you've set your goals, get going!
A GOAL IS A DREAM WITH A DEADLINE.
-Napoleon Hill

PROGRESS PHOTOS
FRONT VIEW

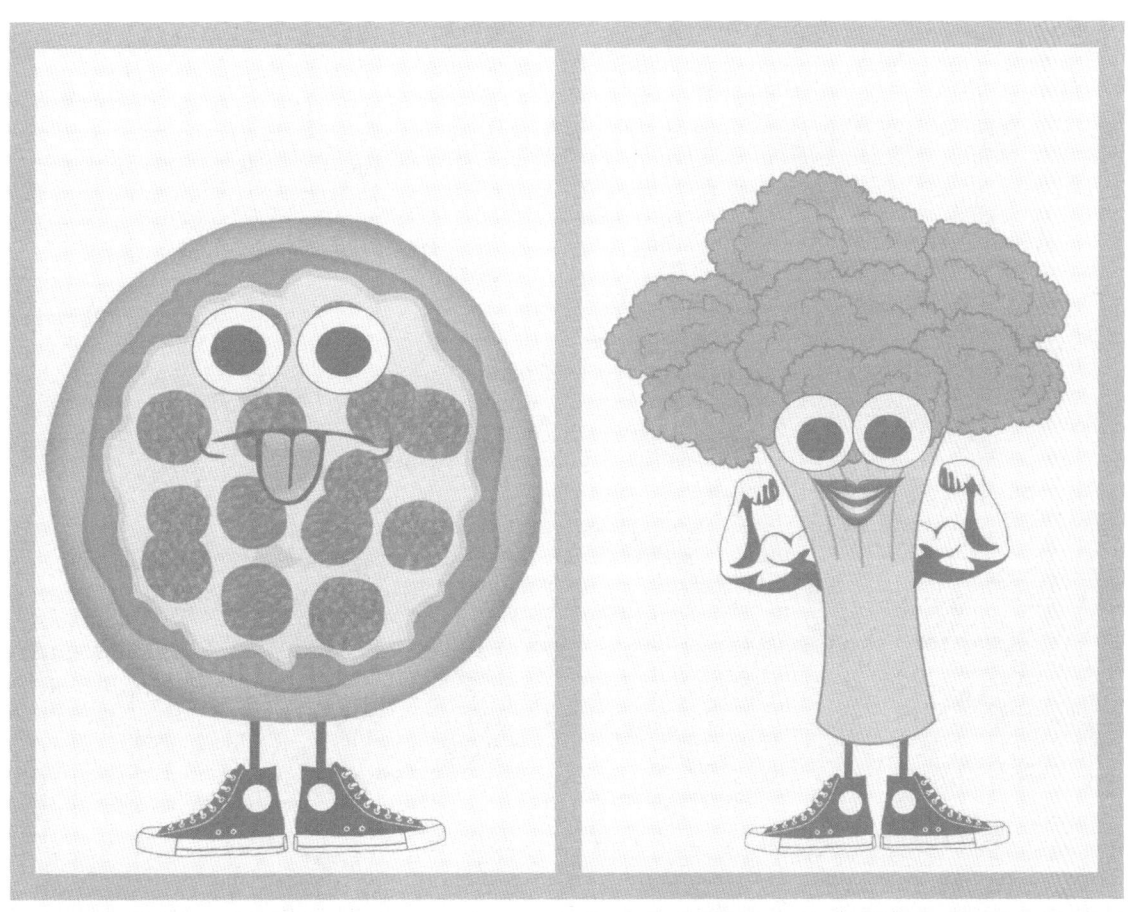

WEEK 1   /   /   **WEEK 13**   /   /

NOTES

PROGRESS PHOTOS
SIDE VIEW

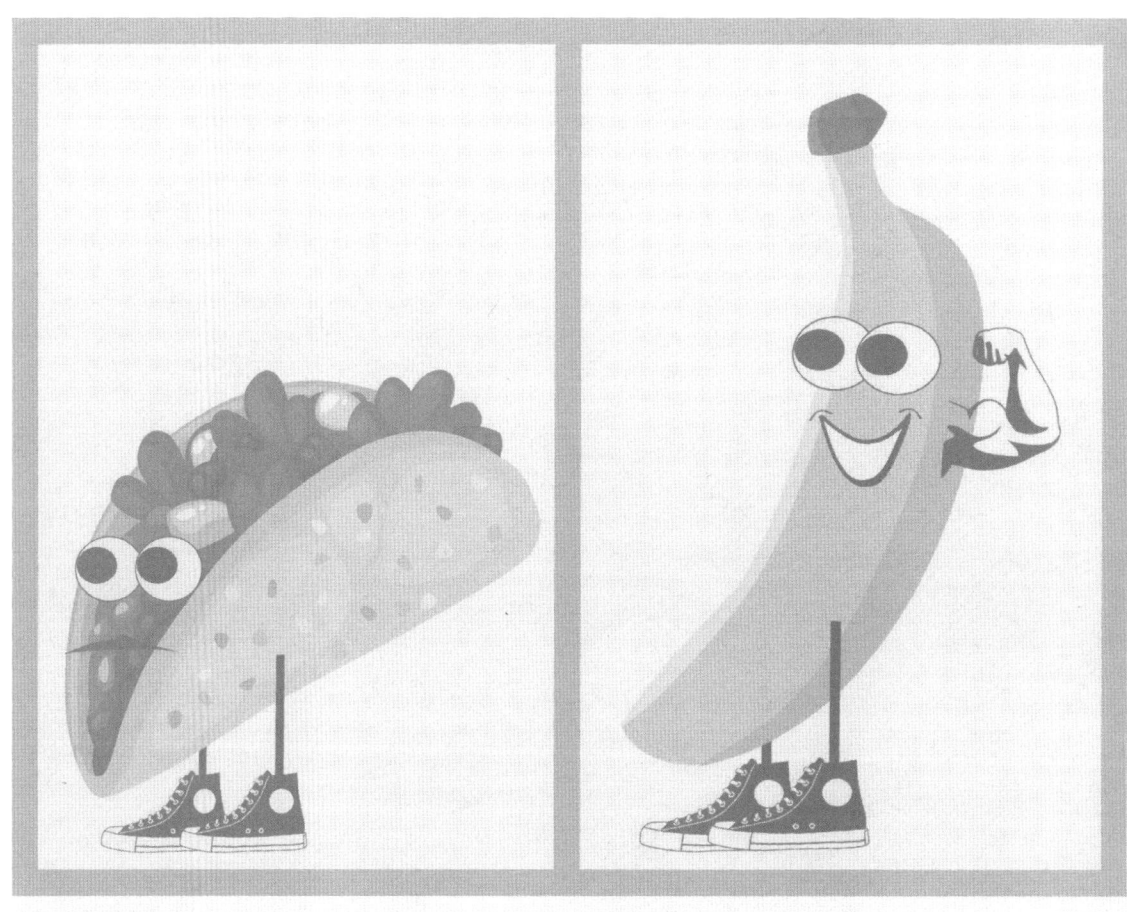

WEEK 1   /   /   **WEEK 13**   /   /

NOTES

PROGRESS PHOTOS
BACK VIEW

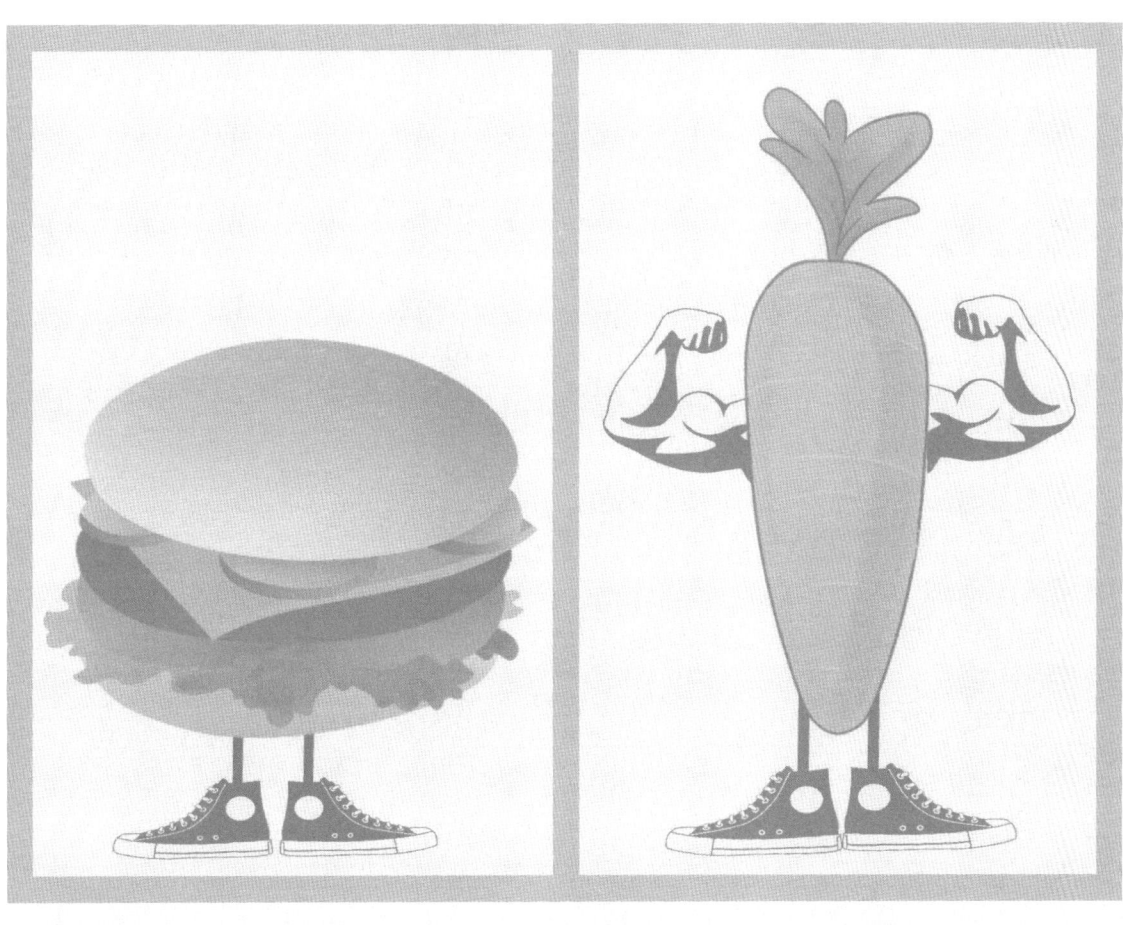

WEEK 1   /   /   **WEEK 13**   /   /

NOTES

MY WEEKLY STATS

	WEEK 1	WEEK 2	WEEK 3	WEEK 4	WEEK 5	WEEK 6
WEIGHT						
BODY FAT %						

MEASUREMENTS

	WEEK 1	WEEK 2	WEEK 3	WEEK 4	WEEK 5	WEEK 6
SHOULDERS						
BUST						
BICEPS						
WAIST						
HIPS						
THIGHS						
CALVES						

ONE REP MAX

	WEEK 1	WEEK 2	WEEK 3	WEEK 4	WEEK 5	WEEK 6
BENCH PRESS						
SQUAT						
DEADLIFT						

OTHER RECORDS

	WEEK 1	WEEK 2	WEEK 3	WEEK 4	WEEK 5	WEEK 6

MY WEEKLY STATS

WEEK 7	WEEK 8	WEEK 9	WEEK 10	WEEK 11	WEEK 12	WEEK 13

MEASUREMENTS

WEEK 7	WEEK 8	WEEK 9	WEEK 10	WEEK 11	WEEK 12	WEEK 13

ONE REP MAX

WEEK 7	WEEK 8	WEEK 9	WEEK 10	WEEK 11	WEEK 12	WEEK 13

OTHER RECORDS

WEEK 7	WEEK 8	WEEK 9	WEEK 10	WEEK 11	WEEK 12	WEEK 13

WOO-HOO! YOU MADE IT!

HYDRATE!

AIM TO CHECK OFF ALL 16 BOXES, ESPECIALLY ON WORKOUT DAYS.

1	= 8 OZ			
2	3	4	5	6
7	8	9	10	11
12	13	14	15	16

FIT TIP:
Take it one meal at a time, one workout at a time. Sometimes "one day at a time" is too overwhelming.

WHAT AM I DOING WELL?

QUOTE OF THE DAY:
A goal properly set is halfway reached.
— Zig Ziglar

HOW CAN I IMPROVE?

WHO CAN I ENCOURAGE OR PRAY FOR TODAY?

1.

MY COMMITMENT TO MYSELF TODAY:

2.

3.

LET IT ALL OUT!

WRITE YOUR FOOD STRUGGLES, MOTIVATION ISSUES, OR EVEN TRACK YOUR SUPPS AND MACROS.

DATE		DAY		TIME		WT	

MOOD — ENERGY LEVEL **1** 2 3 4 5

PROGRAM — PARTNER

MUSCLE FOCUS — LOCATION

STRENGTH TRAINING	S1	S2	S3	S4	S5	SET TYPE	EQUIP-MENT	P.R.

CALS BURNED — END TIME — DURATION

CARDIO	DURATION	DISTANCE	INTENSITY

CALS BURNED — SUPPS USED

HOW WAS MY WORKOUT? **1** 2 3 4 5 6 7 8 9 10

HYDRATE!

☐ = 8 OZ

AIM TO CHECK OFF ALL 16 BOXES, ESPECIALLY ON WORKOUT DAYS.

2	3	4	5	6
7	8	9	10	11
12	13	14	15	16

FIT TIP:
When it gets tough — and it will — keep going.

WHAT AM I DOING WELL?

QUOTE OF THE DAY:
The harder you work, the harder it is to surrender.
— Vince Lombardi

HOW CAN I IMPROVE?

WHO CAN I ENCOURAGE OR PRAY FOR TODAY?

1.

MY COMMITMENT TO MYSELF TODAY:

2.

3.

LET IT ALL OUT!

WRITE YOUR FOOD STRUGGLES, MOTIVATION ISSUES, OR EVEN TRACK YOUR SUPPS AND MACROS.

DATE		DAY		TIME		WT	
MOOD				ENERGY LEVEL		1 2 3 4 5	
PROGRAM				PARTNER			

MUSCLE FOCUS				LOCATION				
STRENGTH TRAINING	S1	S2	S3	S4	S5	SET TYPE	EQUIP-MENT	P.R.

CALS BURNED	END TIME		DURATION	
CARDIO	DURATION	DISTANCE		INTENSITY

CALS BURNED	SUPPS USED	
HOW WAS MY WORKOUT?	1 2 3 4 5 6 7 8 9 10	

HYDRATE!

AIM TO CHECK OFF ALL 16 BOXES, ESPECIALLY ON WORKOUT DAYS.

| 1 | = 8 OZ |

2	3	4	5	6
7	8	9	10	11
12	13	14	15	16

FIT TIP:
On the days when a workout can't happen, focus instead on proper nutrition.

WHAT AM I DOING WELL?

QUOTE OF THE DAY:
Success is how high you bounce when you hit bottom.
— General George Patton

HOW CAN I IMPROVE?

WHO CAN I ENCOURAGE OR PRAY FOR TODAY?

1.

MY COMMITMENT TO MYSELF TODAY:

2.

3.

LET IT ALL OUT!

WRITE YOUR FOOD STRUGGLES, MOTIVATION ISSUES, OR EVEN TRACK YOUR SUPPS AND MACROS.

DATE		DAY		TIME		WT		
MOOD				ENERGY LEVEL		1 2 3 4 5		
PROGRAM				PARTNER				

MUSCLE FOCUS				LOCATION				
STRENGTH TRAINING	S1	S2	S3	S4	S5	SET TYPE	EQUIP-MENT	P.R.

CALS BURNED	END TIME		DURATION	
CARDIO	DURATION	DISTANCE		INTENSITY

CALS BURNED	SUPPS USED	
HOW WAS MY WORKOUT?		1 2 3 4 5 6 7 8 9 10

HYDRATE!

☐ = 8 OZ

AIM TO CHECK OFF ALL 16 BOXES, ESPECIALLY ON WORKOUT DAYS.

1	2	3	4	5	6
	7	8	9	10	11
	12	13	14	15	16

FIT TIP:
When you're around temptation, chew a stick of mint-flavored gum. It will curb cravings and is sure to make those tempting foods taste terrible.

WHAT AM I DOING WELL?

QUOTE OF THE DAY:
The days you work are the best days.
— Georgia O'Keefe

HOW CAN I IMPROVE?

WHO CAN I ENCOURAGE OR PRAY FOR TODAY?

1.

MY COMMITMENT TO MYSELF TODAY:

2.

3.

LET IT ALL OUT!

WRITE YOUR FOOD STRUGGLES, MOTIVATION ISSUES, OR EVEN TRACK YOUR SUPPS AND MACROS.

DATE		DAY		TIME		WT	

MOOD   ENERGY LEVEL **1 2 3 4 5**
PROGRAM   PARTNER

MUSCLE FOCUS					LOCATION			
STRENGTH TRAINING	S1	S2	S3	S4	S5	SET TYPE	EQUIP-MENT	P.R.

CALS BURNED	END TIME		DURATION	
CARDIO	DURATION	DISTANCE		INTENSITY

CALS BURNED	SUPPS USED	
HOW WAS MY WORKOUT?	**1 2 3 4 5 6 7 8 9 10**	

HYDRATE!

AIM TO CHECK OFF ALL 16 BOXES, ESPECIALLY ON WORKOUT DAYS.

| 1 | = 8 OZ |

2	3	4	5	6
7	8	9	10	11
12	13	14	15	16

FIT TIP:
Before you eat, drink 16 ounces of water. It will help fill you up so you don't eat quickly and overindulge.

WHAT AM I DOING WELL?

QUOTE OF THE DAY:
If you can survive disappointment, nothing can beat you.
— Louis C.K.

HOW CAN I IMPROVE?

WHO CAN I ENCOURAGE OR PRAY FOR TODAY?

1.

MY COMMITMENT TO MYSELF TODAY:

2.

3.

LET IT ALL OUT!

WRITE YOUR FOOD STRUGGLES, MOTIVATION ISSUES, OR EVEN TRACK YOUR SUPPS AND MACROS.

DATE		DAY		TIME		WT	
MOOD				ENERGY LEVEL		1 2 3 4 5	
PROGRAM				PARTNER			

MUSCLE FOCUS				LOCATION					
STRENGTH TRAINING	S1	S2	S3	S4	S5	SET TYPE	EQUIPMENT	P.R.

CALS BURNED	END TIME		DURATION	
CARDIO	DURATION	DISTANCE	INTENSITY	

CALS BURNED	SUPPS USED	
HOW WAS MY WORKOUT?	1 2 3 4 5 6 7 8 9 10	

HYDRATE!

☐ = 8 OZ

AIM TO CHECK OFF ALL 16 BOXES, ESPECIALLY ON WORKOUT DAYS.

1	2	3	4	5	6
7	8	9	10	11
12	13	14	15	16

FIT TIP:
Learn your body type! There are three body types: ectomorph, mesomorph, and endomorph. There are unique advantages and challenges for each.

WHAT AM I DOING WELL?

QUOTE OF THE DAY:
We are what we repeatedly do. Excellence, then, is not an act, but a habit.

— Aristotle

HOW CAN I IMPROVE?

WHO CAN I ENCOURAGE OR PRAY FOR TODAY?

1.

MY COMMITMENT TO MYSELF TODAY:

2.

3.

LET IT ALL OUT!

WRITE YOUR FOOD STRUGGLES, MOTIVATION ISSUES, OR EVEN TRACK YOUR SUPPS AND MACROS.

DATE		DAY		TIME		WT	
MOOD				ENERGY LEVEL		1 2 3 4 5	
PROGRAM				PARTNER			

MUSCLE FOCUS				LOCATION				
STRENGTH TRAINING	S1	S2	S3	S4	S5	SET TYPE	EQUIP-MENT	P.R.

CALS BURNED	END TIME		DURATION	
CARDIO	DURATION	DISTANCE		INTENSITY

CALS BURNED	SUPPS USED	
HOW WAS MY WORKOUT?	1 2 3 4 5 6 7 8 9 10	

HYDRATE!

AIM TO CHECK OFF ALL 16 BOXES, ESPECIALLY ON WORKOUT DAYS.

1	= 8 OZ			
2	3	4	5	6
7	8	9	10	11
12	13	14	15	16

FIT TIP:
When you give in to temptation, all is not lost! Immediately pick yourself up and get back on track.

WHAT AM I DOING WELL?

QUOTE OF THE DAY:
You must remain focused on your journey to greatness.
— Les Brown

HOW CAN I IMPROVE?

WHO CAN I ENCOURAGE OR PRAY FOR TODAY?

1.

MY COMMITMENT TO MYSELF TODAY:

2.

3.

LET IT ALL OUT!

WRITE YOUR FOOD STRUGGLES, MOTIVATION ISSUES, OR EVEN TRACK YOUR SUPPS AND MACROS.

IF YOU FAIL TO PLAN...

GOALS FOR THIS WEEK
Specific | **M**easurable | **A**ttainable | **R**ealistic | Time-Bound

Example: I will drink one gallon of water each day this week.

1.

2.

3.

POTIENTIAL ROADBLOCKS	VECTOR CHECK
Anticipate what might throw you off track and plan a solution.	Check each of your written goals and evaluate your progress.
HAZARD: Business luncheon Thurs.	Are you on track to meet your goal?
DETOUR: Protein shake before lunch	
HAZARD:	
	If not, why?
DETOUR:	
HAZARD:	What can you do to get back on track?
DETOUR	
	If you need to modify your goals, do it now!

...YOU ARE PLANNING TO FAIL.

— Benjamin Franklin

MEAL PLANNING
Plan a menu - OR - Write down your meals - OR - Make a grocery list.

SUNDAY

MONDAY

TUESDAY

WEDNESDAY

THURSDAY

FRIDAY
Caution: weekend ahead!

SATURDAY

EXAMPLE A

M1 – oats, protein shake
M2 – whole grain toast & cheese
M3 – scrambled egg white sandwich w/spinach
M4 – carrots & hummus
M5 – chicken, rice, veggies
M6 – pizza (oops!)

EXAMPLE B

– Make turkey chili and protein bars

– Go grocery shopping

– Date Night! Look up restaurant menu

DATE　　　　　　DAY　　　　　　TIME　　　　　　WT
MOOD　　　　　　　　　ENERGY LEVEL　　1　2　3　4　5
PROGRAM　　　　　　　　　　PARTNER

MUSCLE FOCUS					LOCATION			
STRENGTH TRAINING	S1	S2	S3	S4	S5	SET TYPE	EQUIP-MENT	P.R.

CALS BURNED	END TIME		DURATION	
CARDIO	DURATION	DISTANCE		INTENSITY

CALS BURNED	SUPPS USED									
HOW WAS MY WORKOUT?	1	2	3	4	5	6	7	8	9	10

HYDRATE!

AIM TO CHECK OFF ALL 16 BOXES, ESPECIALLY ON WORKOUT DAYS.

[1] = 8 OZ

1	2	3	4	5	6
7	8	9	10	11
12	13	14	15	16

FIT TIP:
Be honest with yourself. When you fail, ask yourself why. Figure out how you can handle it better next time.

WHAT AM I DOING WELL?

QUOTE OF THE DAY:
He gives power to the weak and strength to the powerless.
— Isaiah 40:29

HOW CAN I IMPROVE?

WHO CAN I ENCOURAGE OR PRAY FOR TODAY?

1.

MY COMMITMENT TO MYSELF TODAY:

2.

3.

LET IT ALL OUT!

WRITE YOUR FOOD STRUGGLES, MOTIVATION ISSUES, OR EVEN TRACK YOUR SUPPS AND MACROS.

DATE		DAY		TIME		WT	
MOOD				ENERGY LEVEL		1 2 3 4 5	
PROGRAM				PARTNER			

MUSCLE FOCUS				LOCATION				
STRENGTH TRAINING	S1	S2	S3	S4	S5	SET TYPE	EQUIP-MENT	P.R.

CALS BURNED	END TIME		DURATION	
CARDIO	DURATION	DISTANCE		INTENSITY

CALS BURNED	SUPPS USED	
HOW WAS MY WORKOUT?	1 2 3 4 5 6 7 8 9 10	

HYDRATE!

☐ = 8 OZ

AIM TO CHECK OFF ALL 16 BOXES, ESPECIALLY ON WORKOUT DAYS.

1	2	3	4	5	6
7	8	9	10	11
12	13	14	15	16

FIT TIP:
When possible, work out early so the distractions of the day can't interfere. An early morning workout can energize you and set the tone for your whole day!

WHAT AM I DOING WELL?

QUOTE OF THE DAY:
If somebody tells you no, it doesn't mean you can't do it, it means they can't do it.

— Joel G. Black

HOW CAN I IMPROVE?

WHO CAN I ENCOURAGE OR PRAY FOR TODAY?

1.

MY COMMITMENT TO MYSELF TODAY:

2.

3.

LET IT ALL OUT!

WRITE YOUR FOOD STRUGGLES, MOTIVATION ISSUES, OR EVEN TRACK YOUR SUPPS AND MACROS.

DATE   DAY   TIME   WT
MOOD   ENERGY LEVEL   1 2 3 4 5
PROGRAM   PARTNER

MUSCLE FOCUS				LOCATION				
STRENGTH TRAINING	S1	S2	S3	S4	S5	SET TYPE	EQUIP-MENT	P.R.

CALS BURNED	END TIME		DURATION	
CARDIO	DURATION	DISTANCE		INTENSITY

CALS BURNED	SUPPS USED	
HOW WAS MY WORKOUT?	1 2 3 4 5 6 7 8 9 10	

HYDRATE!

☐ = 8 OZ

AIM TO CHECK OFF ALL 16 BOXES, ESPECIALLY ON WORKOUT DAYS.

1	2	3	4	5	6
7	8	9	10	11
12	13	14	15	16

FIT TIP:
A slow cooker can be your best friend when it comes to meal prep. Find great healthy recipes and meal prep will be painless.

WHAT AM I DOING WELL?

QUOTE OF THE DAY:
Failure is not fatal, but failure to change might be.

— John Wooden

HOW CAN I IMPROVE?

WHO CAN I ENCOURAGE OR PRAY FOR TODAY?

1.

MY COMMITMENT TO MYSELF TODAY:

2.

3.

LET IT ALL OUT!

WRITE YOUR FOOD STRUGGLES, MOTIVATION ISSUES, OR EVEN TRACK YOUR SUPPS AND MACROS.

DATE		DAY		TIME		WT	
MOOD				ENERGY LEVEL		1 2 3 4 5	
PROGRAM				PARTNER			

MUSCLE FOCUS				LOCATION				
STRENGTH TRAINING	S1	S2	S3	S4	S5	SET TYPE	EQUIP-MENT	P.R.

CALS BURNED	END TIME		DURATION	
CARDIO	DURATION	DISTANCE		INTENSITY

CALS BURNED	SUPPS USED	
HOW WAS MY WORKOUT?	1 2 3 4 5 6 7 8 9 10	

HYDRATE!

☐ = 8 OZ

AIM TO CHECK OFF ALL 16 BOXES, ESPECIALLY ON WORKOUT DAYS.

1	2	3	4	5	6
7	8	9	10	11
12	13	14	15	16

FIT TIP:
Find a support system. If you don't have one at home, go online. A great support system is essential to your success.

WHAT AM I DOING WELL?

QUOTE OF THE DAY:
You never achieve success unless you like what you are doing.
— Dale Carnegie

HOW CAN I IMPROVE?

WHO CAN I ENCOURAGE OR PRAY FOR TODAY?

1.

MY COMMITMENT TO MYSELF TODAY:

2.

3.

LET IT ALL OUT!

WRITE YOUR FOOD STRUGGLES, MOTIVATION ISSUES, OR EVEN TRACK YOUR SUPPS AND MACROS.

DATE		DAY		TIME		WT	
MOOD				ENERGY LEVEL		1 2 3 4 5	
PROGRAM				PARTNER			

MUSCLE FOCUS				LOCATION				
STRENGTH TRAINING	S1	S2	S3	S4	S5	SET TYPE	EQUIP-MENT	P.R.

CALS BURNED	END TIME		DURATION	
CARDIO	DURATION	DISTANCE		INTENSITY

CALS BURNED	SUPPS USED	
HOW WAS MY WORKOUT?	1 2 3 4 5 6 7 8 9 10	

HYDRATE!

AIM TO CHECK OFF ALL 16 BOXES, ESPECIALLY ON WORKOUT DAYS.

☐ = 8 OZ

1	2	3	4	5	6
7	8	9	10	11	
12	13	14	15	16	

FIT TIP:
Remember, slow progress is still progress.

WHAT AM I DOING WELL?

QUOTE OF THE DAY:
Stay committed to your decisions, but stay flexible in your approach.
— Anthony Robbins

HOW CAN I IMPROVE?

WHO CAN I ENCOURAGE OR PRAY FOR TODAY?

1.

MY COMMITMENT TO MYSELF TODAY:

2.

3.

LET IT ALL OUT!

WRITE YOUR FOOD STRUGGLES, MOTIVATION ISSUES, OR EVEN TRACK YOUR SUPPS AND MACROS.

DATE		DAY		TIME		WT	
MOOD				ENERGY LEVEL		**1** 2 3 4 5	
PROGRAM				PARTNER			

MUSCLE FOCUS				LOCATION			
STRENGTH TRAINING	S1	S2	S3	S4	S5	SET TYPE	EQUIP-MENT	P.R.

CALS BURNED	END TIME		DURATION	
CARDIO	DURATION	DISTANCE		INTENSITY

CALS BURNED	SUPPS USED	
HOW WAS MY WORKOUT?	1 2 3 4 5 6 7 8 9 10	

HYDRATE!

1 = 8 OZ

AIM TO CHECK OFF ALL 16 BOXES, ESPECIALLY ON WORKOUT DAYS.

1	2	3	4	5	6
	7	8	9	10	11
	12	13	14	15	16

FIT TIP:
Set S.M.A.R.T. goals and reward yourself when you reach them! They should be **S**pecific, **M**easurable, **A**ttainable, **R**ealistic, and **T**ime-Bound.

WHAT AM I DOING WELL?

QUOTE OF THE DAY:
It's always too soon to quit.
- David T. Scoates

HOW CAN I IMPROVE?

WHO CAN I ENCOURAGE OR PRAY FOR TODAY?

1.

MY COMMITMENT TO MYSELF TODAY:

2.

3.

LET IT ALL OUT!

WRITE YOUR FOOD STRUGGLES, MOTIVATION ISSUES, OR EVEN TRACK YOUR SUPPS AND MACROS.

DATE		DAY		TIME		WT	
MOOD				ENERGY LEVEL		1 2 3 4 5	
PROGRAM				PARTNER			

MUSCLE FOCUS			LOCATION					
STRENGTH TRAINING	S1	S2	S3	S4	S5	SET TYPE	EQUIPMENT	P.R.

CALS BURNED	END TIME		DURATION	
CARDIO	DURATION	DISTANCE		INTENSITY

CALS BURNED	SUPPS USED	
HOW WAS MY WORKOUT?		1 2 3 4 5 6 7 8 9 10

HYDRATE!

1 = 8 OZ

AIM TO CHECK OFF ALL 16 BOXES, ESPECIALLY ON WORKOUT DAYS.

2	3	4	5	6
7	8	9	10	11
12	13	14	15	16

FIT TIP:
Fitness does not have to be expensive. Fancy equipment is not required for a great workout! Invest in some resistance bands for an inexpensive workout.

WHAT AM I DOING WELL?

QUOTE OF THE DAY:
Whether you think you can, or you think you can't, you are right.
— Henry Ford

HOW CAN I IMPROVE?

WHO CAN I ENCOURAGE OR PRAY FOR TODAY?

1.

MY COMMITMENT TO MYSELF TODAY:

2.

3.

LET IT ALL OUT!

WRITE YOUR FOOD STRUGGLES, MOTIVATION ISSUES, OR EVEN TRACK YOUR SUPPS AND MACROS.

IF YOU FAIL TO PLAN...

GOALS FOR THIS WEEK
Specific | **M**easurable | **A**ttainable | **R**ealistic | **T**ime-Bound

Example: I will drink one gallon of water each day this week.

1.

2.

3.

POTIENTIAL ROADBLOCKS	VECTOR CHECK
Anticipate what might throw you off track and plan a solution.	Check each of your written goals and evaluate your progress.
HAZARD: Business luncheon Thurs.	Are you on track to meet your goal?
DETOUR: Protein shake before lunch	
HAZARD:	
	If not, why?
DETOUR:	
HAZARD:	What can you do to get back on track?
DETOUR	
	If you need to modify your goals, do it now!

...YOU ARE PLANNING TO FAIL.

— Benjamin Franklin

MEAL PLANNING
Plan a menu - OR - Write down your meals - OR - Make a grocery list.

SUNDAY

MONDAY

TUESDAY

WEDNESDAY

THURSDAY

FRIDAY
Caution: weekend ahead!

SATURDAY

EXAMPLE A

- M1 - oats, protein shake
- M2 - whole grain toast & cheese
- M3 - scrambled egg white sandwich w/spinach
- M4 - carrots & hummus
- M5 - chicken, rice, veggies
- M6 - pizza (oops!)

EXAMPLE B

- Make turkey chili and protein bars

- Go grocery shopping

- Date Night! Look up restaurant menu

DATE		DAY		TIME		WT	
MOOD				ENERGY LEVEL		1 2 3 4 5	
PROGRAM				PARTNER			

MUSCLE FOCUS				LOCATION				
STRENGTH TRAINING	S1	S2	S3	S4	S5	SET TYPE	EQUIPMENT	P.R.

CALS BURNED	END TIME		DURATION	
CARDIO	DURATION	DISTANCE		INTENSITY

CALS BURNED	SUPPS USED	
HOW WAS MY WORKOUT?	1 2 3 4 5 6 7 8 9 10	

HYDRATE!

AIM TO CHECK OFF ALL 16 BOXES, ESPECIALLY ON WORKOUT DAYS.

1 = 8 OZ

1	2	3	4	5	6
7	8	9	10	11	
12	13	14	15	16	

FIT TIP:
When you cook, make extra to freeze so it will be ready in a pinch!

WHAT AM I DOING WELL?

QUOTE OF THE DAY:
The greater the obstacle, the more glory in overcoming it.
— Jean-Baptiste Molière

HOW CAN I IMPROVE?

WHO CAN I ENCOURAGE OR PRAY FOR TODAY?

1.

MY COMMITMENT TO MYSELF TODAY:

2.

3.

LET IT ALL OUT!

WRITE YOUR FOOD STRUGGLES, MOTIVATION ISSUES, OR EVEN TRACK YOUR SUPPS AND MACROS.

DATE   DAY   TIME   WT
MOOD   ENERGY LEVEL 1 2 3 4 5
PROGRAM   PARTNER

MUSCLE FOCUS					LOCATION			
STRENGTH TRAINING	S1	S2	S3	S4	S5	SET TYPE	EQUIP-MENT	P.R.

CALS BURNED	END TIME		DURATION	
CARDIO	DURATION	DISTANCE		INTENSITY

CALS BURNED	SUPPS USED									
HOW WAS MY WORKOUT?	1	2	3	4	5	6	7	8	9	10

HYDRATE!

1 = 8 OZ

AIM TO CHECK OFF ALL 16 BOXES, ESPECIALLY ON WORKOUT DAYS.

2	3	4	5	6
7	8	9	10	11
12	13	14	15	16

FIT TIP:
If you have trigger foods, avoid them! Other foods are fine in moderation.

WHAT AM I DOING WELL?

QUOTE OF THE DAY:
The future is not a gift - it is an achievement.
— Harry Lauder

HOW CAN I IMPROVE?

WHO CAN I ENCOURAGE OR PRAY FOR TODAY?

1.

MY COMMITMENT TO MYSELF TODAY:

2.

3.

LET IT ALL OUT!

WRITE YOUR FOOD STRUGGLES, MOTIVATION ISSUES, OR EVEN TRACK YOUR SUPPS AND MACROS.

DATE		DAY		TIME		WT	
MOOD				ENERGY LEVEL		**1 2 3 4 5**	
PROGRAM				PARTNER			

MUSCLE FOCUS				LOCATION				
STRENGTH TRAINING	S1	S2	S3	S4	S5	SET TYPE	EQUIP-MENT	P.R.

CALS BURNED	END TIME		DURATION	
CARDIO	DURATION	DISTANCE		INTENSITY

CALS BURNED	SUPPS USED	
HOW WAS MY WORKOUT?	**1 2 3 4 5 6 7 8 9 10**	

HYDRATE!

☐ = 8 OZ

AIM TO CHECK OFF ALL 16 BOXES, ESPECIALLY ON WORKOUT DAYS.

1	2	3	4	5	6
	7	8	9	10	11
	12	13	14	15	16

FIT TIP:
Sugar is sneaky and can ruin your progress! It should be limited as much as possible if you're working to get lean.

WHAT AM I DOING WELL?

QUOTE OF THE DAY:
God doesn't require us to succeed, he just requires us to try.
— Mother Teresa

HOW CAN I IMPROVE?

WHO CAN I ENCOURAGE OR PRAY FOR TODAY?

1.

MY COMMITMENT TO MYSELF TODAY:

2.

3.

LET IT ALL OUT!

WRITE YOUR FOOD STRUGGLES, MOTIVATION ISSUES, OR EVEN TRACK YOUR SUPPS AND MACROS.

DATE　　　　　　DAY　　　　　　TIME　　　　　WT
MOOD　　　　　　　　ENERGY LEVEL　**1 2 3 4 5**
PROGRAM　　　　　　　　PARTNER

MUSCLE FOCUS						LOCATION		
STRENGTH TRAINING	S1	S2	S3	S4	S5	SET TYPE	EQUIP-MENT	P.R.

CALS BURNED	END TIME		DURATION	
CARDIO	DURATION	DISTANCE		INTENSITY

CALS BURNED	SUPPS USED									
HOW WAS MY WORKOUT?	1	2	3	4	5	6	7	8	9	10

HYDRATE!

☐ = 8 OZ

AIM TO CHECK OFF ALL 16 BOXES, ESPECIALLY ON WORKOUT DAYS.

1	2	3	4	5	6
7	8	9	10	11
12	13	14	15	16

FIT TIP:
Screw the scale! Remember the scale is just ONE measure of progress, and if you are building muscle, the scale may not budge as your body changes.

WHAT AM I DOING WELL?

QUOTE OF THE DAY:
Success is the ability to go from one failure to another with no loss of enthusiasm.
— Sir Winston Churchill

HOW CAN I IMPROVE?

WHO CAN I ENCOURAGE OR PRAY FOR TODAY?

1.

MY COMMITMENT TO MYSELF TODAY:

2.

3.

LET IT ALL OUT!

WRITE YOUR FOOD STRUGGLES, MOTIVATION ISSUES, OR EVEN TRACK YOUR SUPPS AND MACROS.

DATE　　　　　　DAY　　　　　　TIME　　　　　　WT
MOOD　　　　　　　　　ENERGY LEVEL　　1　2　3　4　5
PROGRAM　　　　　　　　　PARTNER

MUSCLE FOCUS				LOCATION				
STRENGTH TRAINING	S1	S2	S3	S4	S5	SET TYPE	EQUIP-MENT	P.R.

CALS BURNED	END TIME	DURATION
CARDIO DURATION	DISTANCE	INTENSITY

CALS BURNED	SUPPS USED
HOW WAS MY WORKOUT?　1　2　3　4　5　6　7　8　9　10	

HYDRATE!

AIM TO CHECK OFF ALL 16 BOXES, ESPECIALLY ON WORKOUT DAYS.

[1] = 8 OZ

1	2	3	4	5	6
7	8	9	10	11
12	13	14	15	16

FIT TIP:
Don't compare yourself to others; it's a slippery slope that can make you want to quit.

WHAT AM I DOING WELL?

QUOTE OF THE DAY:
It is never too late to be what you might have been.
— George Eliot

HOW CAN I IMPROVE?

WHO CAN I ENCOURAGE OR PRAY FOR TODAY?

1.

MY COMMITMENT TO MYSELF TODAY:

2.

3.

LET IT ALL OUT!

WRITE YOUR FOOD STRUGGLES, MOTIVATION ISSUES, OR EVEN TRACK YOUR SUPPS AND MACROS.

DATE		DAY		TIME		WT	
MOOD				ENERGY LEVEL		1 2 3 4 5	
PROGRAM				PARTNER			

MUSCLE FOCUS				LOCATION				
STRENGTH TRAINING	S1	S2	S3	S4	S5	SET TYPE	EQUIP-MENT	P.R.

CALS BURNED	END TIME		DURATION	
CARDIO	DURATION	DISTANCE		INTENSITY

CALS BURNED	SUPPS USED	
HOW WAS MY WORKOUT?	1 2 3 4 5 6 7 8 9 10	

HYDRATE!

AIM TO CHECK OFF ALL 16 BOXES, ESPECIALLY ON WORKOUT DAYS.

1	= 8 OZ			
2	3	4	5	6
7	8	9	10	11
12	13	14	15	16

FIT TIP:
Food is not the enemy. Building muscle means eating MORE! Don't be afraid of food.

WHAT AM I DOING WELL?

QUOTE OF THE DAY:
Being defeated is often a temporary condition. Giving up is what makes it permanent.
— Marilyn vos Savant

HOW CAN I IMPROVE?

WHO CAN I ENCOURAGE OR PRAY FOR TODAY?

1.

MY COMMITMENT TO MYSELF TODAY:

2.

3.

LET IT ALL OUT!

WRITE YOUR FOOD STRUGGLES, MOTIVATION ISSUES, OR EVEN TRACK YOUR SUPPS AND MACROS.

DATE   DAY   TIME   WT
MOOD   ENERGY LEVEL   1 2 3 4 5
PROGRAM   PARTNER

MUSCLE FOCUS						LOCATION		
STRENGTH TRAINING	S1	S2	S3	S4	S5	SET TYPE	EQUIP-MENT	P.R.

CALS BURNED	END TIME	DURATION
CARDIO DURATION	DISTANCE	INTENSITY

CALS BURNED	SUPPS USED	
HOW WAS MY WORKOUT?	1 2 3 4 5 6 7 8 9 10	

HYDRATE!

AIM TO CHECK OFF ALL 16 BOXES, ESPECIALLY ON WORKOUT DAYS.

| 1 | = 8 OZ |

1	2	3	4	5	6
7	8	9	10	11
12	13	14	15	16

FIT TIP:
You may not enjoy cardio, but it is important for fat loss, as well as overall health. Try HIIT cardio to switch things up!

WHAT AM I DOING WELL?

QUOTE OF THE DAY:
She believed she could, so she did.
— R.S. Grey

HOW CAN I IMPROVE?

WHO CAN I ENCOURAGE OR PRAY FOR TODAY?

1.

MY COMMITMENT TO MYSELF TODAY:

2.

3.

LET IT ALL OUT!

WRITE YOUR FOOD STRUGGLES, MOTIVATION ISSUES, OR EVEN TRACK YOUR SUPPS AND MACROS.

IF YOU FAIL TO PLAN...

GOALS FOR THIS WEEK
Specific | **M**easurable | **A**ttainable | **R**ealistic | **T**ime-Bound

Example: I will drink one gallon of water each day this week.

1.

2.

3.

POTIENTIAL ROADBLOCKS	VECTOR CHECK
Anticipate what might throw you off track and plan a solution.	Check each of your written goals and evaluate your progress.
HAZARD: Business luncheon Thurs.	Are you on track to meet your goal?
DETOUR: Protein shake before lunch	
HAZARD:	
	If not, why?
DETOUR:	
HAZARD:	What can you do to get back on track?
DETOUR	
	If you need to modify your goals, do it now!

...YOU ARE PLANNING TO FAIL.

— Benjamin Franklin

MEAL PLANNING
Plan a menu - OR - Write down your meals - OR - Make a grocery list.

SUNDAY

MONDAY

TUESDAY

WEDNESDAY

THURSDAY

FRIDAY
Caution: weekend ahead!

SATURDAY

EXAMPLE A

M1 - oats, protein shake
M2 - whole grain toast & cheese
M3 - scrambled egg white sandwich w/spinach
M4 - carrots & hummus
M5 - chicken, rice, veggies
M6 - pizza (oops!)

EXAMPLE B

- Make turkey chili and protein bars
- Go grocery shopping
- Date Night! Look up restaurant menu

DATE		DAY		TIME		WT	
MOOD				ENERGY LEVEL	1 2 3 4 5		
PROGRAM				PARTNER			

MUSCLE FOCUS				LOCATION			
STRENGTH TRAINING	S1	S2	S3	S4	S5	SET TYPE	EQUIP-MENT	P.R.

CALS BURNED	END TIME		DURATION	
CARDIO	DURATION	DISTANCE		INTENSITY

CALS BURNED	SUPPS USED	
HOW WAS MY WORKOUT?	1 2 3 4 5 6 7 8 9 10	

HYDRATE!

AIM TO CHECK OFF ALL 16 BOXES, ESPECIALLY ON WORKOUT DAYS.

1	= 8 OZ			
2	3	4	5	6
7	8	9	10	11
12	13	14	15	16

FIT TIP:
Calorie cycle to give your body what it needs. Consume fewer on rest days, and more on heavy lifting days.

WHAT AM I DOING WELL?

QUOTE OF THE DAY:
Feel the fear and do it anyway.
— Susan Jeffers

HOW CAN I IMPROVE?

WHO CAN I ENCOURAGE OR PRAY FOR TODAY?

1.

MY COMMITMENT TO MYSELF TODAY:

2.

3.

LET IT ALL OUT!

WRITE YOUR FOOD STRUGGLES, MOTIVATION ISSUES, OR EVEN TRACK YOUR SUPPS AND MACROS.

DATE		DAY		TIME		WT	
MOOD				ENERGY LEVEL		1 2 3 4 5	
PROGRAM				PARTNER			

MUSCLE FOCUS				LOCATION				
STRENGTH TRAINING	S1	S2	S3	S4	S5	SET TYPE	EQUIP-MENT	P.R.

CALS BURNED	END TIME		DURATION	
CARDIO	DURATION	DISTANCE		INTENSITY

CALS BURNED	SUPPS USED	
HOW WAS MY WORKOUT?	1 2 3 4 5 6 7 8 9 10	

HYDRATE!

AIM TO CHECK OFF ALL 16 BOXES, ESPECIALLY ON WORKOUT DAYS.

☐1 = 8 OZ

2	3	4	5	6
7	8	9	10	11
12	13	14	15	16

FIT TIP:
"All things in moderation" isn't always the best advice. Sometimes moderation leads to overindulgence.

WHAT AM I DOING WELL?

QUOTE OF THE DAY:
The noblest search is the search for excellence.
— Lyndon B. Johnson

HOW CAN I IMPROVE?

WHO CAN I ENCOURAGE OR PRAY FOR TODAY?

1.

MY COMMITMENT TO MYSELF TODAY:

2.

3.

LET IT ALL OUT!

WRITE YOUR FOOD STRUGGLES, MOTIVATION ISSUES, OR EVEN TRACK YOUR SUPPS AND MACROS.

DATE		DAY		TIME		WT	
MOOD				ENERGY LEVEL		1 2 3 4 5	
PROGRAM				PARTNER			

MUSCLE FOCUS				LOCATION				
STRENGTH TRAINING	S1	S2	S3	S4	S5	SET TYPE	EQUIPMENT	P.R.

CALS BURNED	END TIME		DURATION	
CARDIO	DURATION	DISTANCE		INTENSITY

CALS BURNED	SUPPS USED	
HOW WAS MY WORKOUT?	1 2 3 4 5 6 7 8 9 10	

HYDRATE!

AIM TO CHECK OFF ALL 16 BOXES, ESPECIALLY ON WORKOUT DAYS.

[1] = 8 OZ

2	3	4	5	6
7	8	9	10	11
12	13	14	15	16

FIT TIP:
If you are tired of starting over, stop quitting!

WHAT AM I DOING WELL?

QUOTE OF THE DAY:
It always seems impossible until it's done.
— Nelson Mandela

HOW CAN I IMPROVE?

WHO CAN I ENCOURAGE OR PRAY FOR TODAY?

1.

MY COMMITMENT TO MYSELF TODAY:

2.

3.

LET IT ALL OUT!

WRITE YOUR FOOD STRUGGLES, MOTIVATION ISSUES, OR EVEN TRACK YOUR SUPPS AND MACROS.

DATE		DAY		TIME		WT	
MOOD				ENERGY LEVEL		1 2 3 4 5	
PROGRAM				PARTNER			

MUSCLE FOCUS				LOCATION				
STRENGTH TRAINING	S1	S2	S3	S4	S5	SET TYPE	EQUIPMENT	P.R.

CALS BURNED	END TIME	DURATION	
CARDIO	DURATION	DISTANCE	INTENSITY

CALS BURNED	SUPPS USED	
HOW WAS MY WORKOUT?		1 2 3 4 5 6 7 8 9 10

HYDRATE!

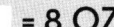 = 8 OZ

AIM TO CHECK OFF ALL 16 BOXES, ESPECIALLY ON WORKOUT DAYS.

FIT TIP:
When you are questioned about your fit lifestyle, take that opportunity to explain to others exactly what you're doing. Maybe they'll join you!

WHAT AM I DOING WELL?

QUOTE OF THE DAY:
A year from now you may wish you had started today.
- Karen Lamb

HOW CAN I IMPROVE?

WHO CAN I ENCOURAGE OR PRAY FOR TODAY?

1.

MY COMMITMENT TO MYSELF TODAY:

2.

3.

LET IT ALL OUT!

WRITE YOUR FOOD STRUGGLES, MOTIVATION ISSUES, OR EVEN TRACK YOUR SUPPS AND MACROS.

DATE		DAY		TIME		WT	
MOOD				ENERGY LEVEL		1 2 3 4 5	
PROGRAM				PARTNER			

MUSCLE FOCUS				LOCATION					
STRENGTH TRAINING	S1	S2	S3	S4	S5	SET TYPE	EQUIP-MENT	P.R.

CALS BURNED	END TIME		DURATION	
CARDIO	DURATION	DISTANCE		INTENSITY

CALS BURNED	SUPPS USED	
HOW WAS MY WORKOUT?	1 2 3 4 5 6 7 8 9 10	

HYDRATE!

AIM TO CHECK OFF ALL 16 BOXES, ESPECIALLY ON WORKOUT DAYS.

1 = 8 OZ

1	2	3	4	5	6
7	8	9	10	11	
12	13	14	15	16	

FIT TIP:
Lack of planning often leads to poor decisions. Take the time to make a plan, and develop the discipline to stick with it.

WHAT AM I DOING WELL?

QUOTE OF THE DAY:
Our intention creates our reality.
— Wayne Dyer

HOW CAN I IMPROVE?

WHO CAN I ENCOURAGE OR PRAY FOR TODAY?

1.

MY COMMITMENT TO MYSELF TODAY:

2.

3.

LET IT ALL OUT!

WRITE YOUR FOOD STRUGGLES, MOTIVATION ISSUES, OR EVEN TRACK YOUR SUPPS AND MACROS.

DATE		DAY		TIME		WT	
MOOD				ENERGY LEVEL		1 2 3 4 5	
PROGRAM				PARTNER			

MUSCLE FOCUS				LOCATION				
STRENGTH TRAINING	S1	S2	S3	S4	S5	SET TYPE	EQUIPMENT	P.R.

CALS BURNED	END TIME		DURATION	
CARDIO	DURATION	DISTANCE		INTENSITY

CALS BURNED	SUPPS USED	
HOW WAS MY WORKOUT?	1 2 3 4 5 6 7 8 9 10	

HYDRATE!

AIM TO CHECK OFF ALL 16 BOXES, ESPECIALLY ON WORKOUT DAYS.

1	= 8 OZ			
2	3	4	5	6
7	8	9	10	11
12	13	14	15	16

FIT TIP:
Challenge yourself to try something new, whether it's a new food (quinoa!) or an intimidating exercise (box jumps!).

WHAT AM I DOING WELL?

QUOTE OF THE DAY:
Nothing worth having was ever achieved without effort.
— Theodore Roosevelt

HOW CAN I IMPROVE?

WHO CAN I ENCOURAGE OR PRAY FOR TODAY?

1.

MY COMMITMENT TO MYSELF TODAY:

2.

3.

LET IT ALL OUT!

WRITE YOUR FOOD STRUGGLES, MOTIVATION ISSUES, OR EVEN TRACK YOUR SUPPS AND MACROS.

DATE		DAY		TIME		WT	
MOOD				ENERGY LEVEL		1 2 3 4 5	
PROGRAM				PARTNER			

MUSCLE FOCUS				LOCATION				
STRENGTH TRAINING	S1	S2	S3	S4	S5	SET TYPE	EQUIP-MENT	P.R.

CALS BURNED	END TIME		DURATION	
CARDIO	DURATION	DISTANCE		INTENSITY

CALS BURNED	SUPPS USED	
HOW WAS MY WORKOUT?	1 2 3 4 5 6 7 8 9 10	

HYDRATE!

▢ = 8 OZ

AIM TO CHECK OFF ALL 16 BOXES, ESPECIALLY ON WORKOUT DAYS.

1	2	3	4	5	6
7	8	9	10	11
12	13	14	15	16

FIT TIP:
If you hire a personal trainer, do your research. Choosing the wrong one can have a severe impact on your mental and physical health.

WHAT AM I DOING WELL?

QUOTE OF THE DAY:
Success isn't a result of spontaneous combustion. You must set yourself on fire.
— Arnold H. Glasow

HOW CAN I IMPROVE?

WHO CAN I ENCOURAGE OR PRAY FOR TODAY?

1.

MY COMMITMENT TO MYSELF TODAY:

2.

3.

LET IT ALL OUT!

WRITE YOUR FOOD STRUGGLES, MOTIVATION ISSUES, OR EVEN TRACK YOUR SUPPS AND MACROS.

IF YOU FAIL TO PLAN...

GOALS FOR THIS WEEK
Specific | **M**easurable | **A**ttainable | **R**ealistic | **T**ime-Bound

Example: I will drink one gallon of water each day this week.

1.

2.

3.

POTIENTIAL ROADBLOCKS	VECTOR CHECK
Anticipate what might throw you off track and plan a solution.	Check each of your written goals and evaluate your progress.
HAZARD: Business luncheon Thurs.	Are you on track to meet your goal?
DETOUR: Protein shake before lunch	
HAZARD:	
	If not, why?
DETOUR:	
HAZARD:	What can you do to get back on track?
DETOUR	
	If you need to modify your goals, do it now!

...YOU ARE PLANNING TO FAIL.

— Benjamin Franklin

MEAL PLANNING
Plan a menu - OR - Write down your meals - OR - Make a grocery list.

SUNDAY

MONDAY

TUESDAY

WEDNESDAY

THURSDAY

FRIDAY
Caution: weekend ahead!

SATURDAY

EXAMPLE A

- M1 - oats, protein shake
- M2 - whole grain toast & cheese
- M3 - scrambled egg white sandwich w/spinach
- M4 - carrots & hummus
- M5 - chicken, rice, veggies
- M6 - pizza (oops!)

EXAMPLE B

- Make turkey chili and protein bars
- Go grocery shopping
- Date Night! Look up restaurant menu

DATE		DAY		TIME		WT	
MOOD				ENERGY LEVEL		1 2 3 4 5	
PROGRAM				PARTNER			

MUSCLE FOCUS				LOCATION				
STRENGTH TRAINING	S1	S2	S3	S4	S5	SET TYPE	EQUIPMENT	P.R.

CALS BURNED	END TIME		DURATION	
CARDIO	DURATION	DISTANCE		INTENSITY

CALS BURNED	SUPPS USED	
HOW WAS MY WORKOUT?	1 2 3 4 5 6 7 8 9 10	

HYDRATE!

1 = 8 OZ

AIM TO CHECK OFF ALL 16 BOXES, ESPECIALLY ON WORKOUT DAYS.

2	3	4	5	6
7	8	9	10	11
12	13	14	15	16

FIT TIP:
No one wants to take "before" photos. Take them, anyway. You'll be glad you did.

WHAT AM I DOING WELL?

QUOTE OF THE DAY:
I hope that I may always desire more than I can accomplish.
— Michelangelo

HOW CAN I IMPROVE?

WHO CAN I ENCOURAGE OR PRAY FOR TODAY?

1.

MY COMMITMENT TO MYSELF TODAY:

2.

3.

LET IT ALL OUT!

WRITE YOUR FOOD STRUGGLES, MOTIVATION ISSUES, OR EVEN TRACK YOUR SUPPS AND MACROS.

DATE DAY TIME WT
MOOD ENERGY LEVEL **1 2 3 4 5**
PROGRAM PARTNER

MUSCLE FOCUS			LOCATION					
STRENGTH TRAINING	S1	S2	S3	S4	S5	SET TYPE	EQUIP-MENT	P.R.

CALS BURNED	END TIME		DURATION	
CARDIO	DURATION	DISTANCE		INTENSITY

CALS BURNED	SUPPS USED	
HOW WAS MY WORKOUT?	**1 2 3 4 5 6 7 8 9 10**	

HYDRATE!

☐ = 8 OZ

AIM TO CHECK OFF ALL 16 BOXES, ESPECIALLY ON WORKOUT DAYS.

1	2	3	4	5	6
	7	8	9	10	11
	12	13	14	15	16

FIT TIP:
Remember that everyone was once a beginner.

WHAT AM I DOING WELL?

QUOTE OF THE DAY:
Let our advance worrying become advance thinking and planning.
— Sir Winston Churchill

HOW CAN I IMPROVE?

WHO CAN I ENCOURAGE OR PRAY FOR TODAY?

1.

MY COMMITMENT TO MYSELF TODAY:

2.

3.

LET IT ALL OUT!

WRITE YOUR FOOD STRUGGLES, MOTIVATION ISSUES, OR EVEN TRACK YOUR SUPPS AND MACROS.

DATE DAY TIME WT
MOOD ENERGY LEVEL **1** 2 3 4 5
PROGRAM PARTNER

MUSCLE FOCUS			LOCATION					
STRENGTH TRAINING	S1	S2	S3	S4	S5	SET TYPE	EQUIPMENT	P.R.

CALS BURNED	END TIME		DURATION	
CARDIO	DURATION	DISTANCE		INTENSITY

CALS BURNED	SUPPS USED									
HOW WAS MY WORKOUT?	1	2	3	4	5	6	7	8	9	10

HYDRATE!

AIM TO CHECK OFF ALL 16 BOXES, ESPECIALLY ON WORKOUT DAYS.

1 = 8 OZ

2	3	4	5	6
7	8	9	10	11
12	13	14	15	16

FIT TIP:
Each time you take progress pics, wear the same clothing and take photos at the same time of day.

WHAT AM I DOING WELL?

QUOTE OF THE DAY:
You are what you think about all day long.
— Robert H. Schuller

HOW CAN I IMPROVE?

WHO CAN I ENCOURAGE OR PRAY FOR TODAY?

1.

MY COMMITMENT TO MYSELF TODAY:

2.

3.

LET IT ALL OUT!

WRITE YOUR FOOD STRUGGLES, MOTIVATION ISSUES, OR EVEN TRACK YOUR SUPPS AND MACROS.

DATE		DAY		TIME		WT	
MOOD			ENERGY LEVEL		1 2 3 4 5		
PROGRAM				PARTNER			

MUSCLE FOCUS				LOCATION			
STRENGTH TRAINING	S1	S2	S3	S4	S5	SET TYPE	EQUIP-MENT	P.R.

CALS BURNED	END TIME		DURATION	
CARDIO	DURATION	DISTANCE		INTENSITY

CALS BURNED	SUPPS USED	
HOW WAS MY WORKOUT?	1 2 3 4 5 6 7 8 9 10	

HYDRATE!

☐ = 8 OZ

AIM TO CHECK OFF ALL 16 BOXES, ESPECIALLY ON WORKOUT DAYS.

1	2	3	4	5	6
7	8	9	10	11
12	13	14	15	16

FIT TIP:
Starting is the hardest part. Once you build momentum, it becomes habit and gets easier.

WHAT AM I DOING WELL?

QUOTE OF THE DAY:
To live is the rarest thing in the world, most people just exist.
— Oscar Wilde

HOW CAN I IMPROVE?

WHO CAN I ENCOURAGE OR PRAY FOR TODAY?

1.

MY COMMITMENT TO MYSELF TODAY:

2.

3.

LET IT ALL OUT!

WRITE YOUR FOOD STRUGGLES, MOTIVATION ISSUES, OR EVEN TRACK YOUR SUPPS AND MACROS.

DATE		DAY		TIME		WT	
MOOD				ENERGY LEVEL		1 2 3 4 5	
PROGRAM				PARTNER			

MUSCLE FOCUS				LOCATION			
STRENGTH TRAINING	S1	S2	S3	S4	S5	SET TYPE	EQUIPMENT	P.R.

CALS BURNED	END TIME		DURATION	
CARDIO	DURATION	DISTANCE		INTENSITY

CALS BURNED	SUPPS USED	
HOW WAS MY WORKOUT?	1 2 3 4 5 6 7 8 9 10	

HYDRATE!

1 = 8 OZ

AIM TO CHECK OFF ALL 16 BOXES, ESPECIALLY ON WORKOUT DAYS.

2	3	4	5	6
7	8	9	10	11
12	13	14	15	16

FIT TIP:
You'll never reach your goals if you don't believe you can.

WHAT AM I DOING WELL?

QUOTE OF THE DAY:
Act as if you have already achieved your goal and it is yours.
— Dr. Robert Anthony

HOW CAN I IMPROVE?

WHO CAN I ENCOURAGE OR PRAY FOR TODAY?

1.

MY COMMITMENT TO MYSELF TODAY:

2.

3.

LET IT ALL OUT!

WRITE YOUR FOOD STRUGGLES, MOTIVATION ISSUES, OR EVEN TRACK YOUR SUPPS AND MACROS.

DATE		DAY		TIME		WT	
MOOD			ENERGY LEVEL		1 2 3 4 5		
PROGRAM				PARTNER			

MUSCLE FOCUS				LOCATION			
STRENGTH TRAINING	S1	S2	S3	S4	S5	SET TYPE	EQUIP-MENT	P.R.

CALS BURNED	END TIME		DURATION	
CARDIO	DURATION	DISTANCE		INTENSITY

CALS BURNED	SUPPS USED	
HOW WAS MY WORKOUT?	1 2 3 4 5 6 7 8 9 10	

HYDRATE!

AIM TO CHECK OFF ALL 16 BOXES, ESPECIALLY ON WORKOUT DAYS.

| 1 | = 8 OZ |

2	3	4	5	6
7	8	9	10	11
12	13	14	15	16

FIT TIP:

God created you for great things. He's got your back, and that is all that matters.

WHAT AM I DOING WELL?

QUOTE OF THE DAY:

Don't let what you cannot do interfere with what you can do.

— John Wooden

HOW CAN I IMPROVE?

WHO CAN I ENCOURAGE OR PRAY FOR TODAY?

1.

MY COMMITMENT TO MYSELF TODAY:

2.

3.

LET IT ALL OUT!

WRITE YOUR FOOD STRUGGLES, MOTIVATION ISSUES, OR EVEN TRACK YOUR SUPPS AND MACROS.

DATE   DAY   TIME   WT
MOOD   ENERGY LEVEL   1 2 3 4 5
PROGRAM   PARTNER

MUSCLE FOCUS			LOCATION					
STRENGTH TRAINING	S1	S2	S3	S4	S5	SET TYPE	EQUIP-MENT	P.R.

CALS BURNED	END TIME		DURATION	
CARDIO	DURATION	DISTANCE		INTENSITY

CALS BURNED	SUPPS USED									
HOW WAS MY WORKOUT?	1	2	3	4	5	6	7	8	9	10

HYDRATE!

AIM TO CHECK OFF ALL 16 BOXES, ESPECIALLY ON WORKOUT DAYS.

1	= 8 OZ			
2	3	4	5	6
7	8	9	10	11
12	13	14	15	16

FIT TIP:
You are special, you are the only you, and you are worth the effort it takes.

WHAT AM I DOING WELL?

QUOTE OF THE DAY:
She is energetic and strong, a hard worker.
— Proverbs 31:17

HOW CAN I IMPROVE?

WHO CAN I ENCOURAGE OR PRAY FOR TODAY?

1.

MY COMMITMENT TO MYSELF TODAY:

2.

3.

LET IT ALL OUT!

WRITE YOUR FOOD STRUGGLES, MOTIVATION ISSUES, OR EVEN TRACK YOUR SUPPS AND MACROS.

IF YOU FAIL TO PLAN...

GOALS FOR THIS WEEK
Specific | **M**easurable | **A**ttainable | **R**ealistic | **T**ime-Bound

Example: I will drink one gallon of water each day this week.

1.

2.

3.

POTIENTIAL ROADBLOCKS	VECTOR CHECK
Anticipate what might throw you off track and plan a solution.	Check each of your written goals and evaluate your progress.
HAZARD: Business luncheon Thurs.	Are you on track to meet your goal?
DETOUR: Protein shake before lunch	
HAZARD:	
	If not, why?
DETOUR:	
HAZARD:	What can you do to get back on track?
DETOUR	
	If you need to modify your goals, do it now!

… YOU ARE PLANNING TO FAIL.

— Benjamin Franklin

MEAL PLANNING

Plan a menu - OR - Write down your meals - OR - Make a grocery list.

SUNDAY

MONDAY

TUESDAY

WEDNESDAY

THURSDAY

FRIDAY
Caution: weekend ahead!

SATURDAY

EXAMPLE A

- M1 – oats, protein shake
- M2 – whole grain toast & cheese
- M3 – scrambled egg white sandwich w/spinach
- M4 – carrots & hummus
- M5 – chicken, rice, veggies
- M6 – pizza (oops!)

EXAMPLE B

- Make turkey chili and protein bars
- Go grocery shopping
- Date Night! Look up restaurant menu

DATE		DAY		TIME		WT	
MOOD				ENERGY LEVEL		1 2 3 4 5	
PROGRAM				PARTNER			

MUSCLE FOCUS				LOCATION					
STRENGTH TRAINING	S1	S2	S3	S4	S5	SET TYPE	EQUIP-MENT	P.R.

CALS BURNED	END TIME		DURATION	
CARDIO	DURATION	DISTANCE	INTENSITY	

CALS BURNED	SUPPS USED	
HOW WAS MY WORKOUT?	1 2 3 4 5 6 7 8 9 10	

HYDRATE!

AIM TO CHECK OFF ALL 16 BOXES, ESPECIALLY ON WORKOUT DAYS.

1	= 8 OZ			
2	3	4	5	6
7	8	9	10	11
12	13	14	15	16

FIT TIP:
Get with the program! There are many great FREE fitness programs available online to help you get started.

WHAT AM I DOING WELL?

QUOTE OF THE DAY:
The great pleasure in life is doing what people say you cannot do.
— Walter Bagehot

HOW CAN I IMPROVE?

WHO CAN I ENCOURAGE OR PRAY FOR TODAY?

1.

MY COMMITMENT TO MYSELF TODAY:

2.

3.

LET IT ALL OUT!

WRITE YOUR FOOD STRUGGLES, MOTIVATION ISSUES, OR EVEN TRACK YOUR SUPPS AND MACROS.

DATE		DAY		TIME		WT	
MOOD				ENERGY LEVEL		**1** 2 3 4 5	
PROGRAM				PARTNER			

MUSCLE FOCUS				LOCATION				
STRENGTH TRAINING	S1	S2	S3	S4	S5	SET TYPE	EQUIP-MENT	P.R.

CALS BURNED	END TIME		DURATION	
CARDIO	DURATION	DISTANCE		INTENSITY

CALS BURNED	SUPPS USED	
HOW WAS MY WORKOUT?	1 2 3 4 5 6 7 8 9 10	

HYDRATE!

AIM TO CHECK OFF ALL 16 BOXES, ESPECIALLY ON WORKOUT DAYS.

☐ = 8 OZ

2	3	4	5	6
7	8	9	10	11
12	13	14	15	16

FIT TIP:
New music on your playlist can put some pep in your step and add some extra intensity to your workout sessions.

WHAT AM I DOING WELL?

QUOTE OF THE DAY:
Giving up is the ultimate tragedy.
— Robert J. Donavan

HOW CAN I IMPROVE?

WHO CAN I ENCOURAGE OR PRAY FOR TODAY?

1.

MY COMMITMENT TO MYSELF TODAY:

2.

3.

LET IT ALL OUT!

WRITE YOUR FOOD STRUGGLES, MOTIVATION ISSUES, OR EVEN TRACK YOUR SUPPS AND MACROS.

DATE		DAY		TIME		WT	
MOOD				ENERGY LEVEL		1 2 3 4 5	
PROGRAM				PARTNER			

MUSCLE FOCUS				LOCATION					
STRENGTH TRAINING	S1	S2	S3	S4	S5	SET TYPE	EQUIP-MENT	P.R.

CALS BURNED	END TIME	DURATION

CARDIO	DURATION	DISTANCE	INTENSITY

CALS BURNED	SUPPS USED

HOW WAS MY WORKOUT?	1 2 3 4 5 6 7 8 9 10

HYDRATE!

AIM TO CHECK OFF ALL 16 BOXES, ESPECIALLY ON WORKOUT DAYS.

☐ = 8 OZ

1	2	3	4	5	6
7	8	9	10	11	
12	13	14	15	16	

FIT TIP:
Before you make decisions about your nutrition or workouts, stop to ask yourself if you'll be proud of that decision tomorrow.

WHAT AM I DOING WELL?

QUOTE OF THE DAY:
Action is the foundational key to all success.
— Pablo Picasso

HOW CAN I IMPROVE?

WHO CAN I ENCOURAGE OR PRAY FOR TODAY?

1.

MY COMMITMENT TO MYSELF TODAY:

2.

3.

LET IT ALL OUT!

WRITE YOUR FOOD STRUGGLES, MOTIVATION ISSUES, OR EVEN TRACK YOUR SUPPS AND MACROS.

DATE   DAY   TIME   WT
MOOD   ENERGY LEVEL   1 2 3 4 5
PROGRAM   PARTNER

MUSCLE FOCUS						LOCATION		
STRENGTH TRAINING	S1	S2	S3	S4	S5	SET TYPE	EQUIP-MENT	P.R.

CALS BURNED	END TIME		DURATION	
CARDIO	DURATION	DISTANCE		INTENSITY

CALS BURNED	SUPPS USED									
HOW WAS MY WORKOUT?	1	2	3	4	5	6	7	8	9	10

HYDRATE!

AIM TO CHECK OFF ALL 16 BOXES, ESPECIALLY ON WORKOUT DAYS.

1 = 8 OZ

1	2	3	4	5	6
7	8	9	10	11	
12	13	14	15	16	

FIT TIP:
Write down your goals. If you don't write them down, they are just dreams.

WHAT AM I DOING WELL?

QUOTE OF THE DAY:
The best thing about the future is that it only comes one day at a time.
— Abraham Lincoln

HOW CAN I IMPROVE?

WHO CAN I ENCOURAGE OR PRAY FOR TODAY?

1.

MY COMMITMENT TO MYSELF TODAY:

2.

3.

LET IT ALL OUT!

WRITE YOUR FOOD STRUGGLES, MOTIVATION ISSUES, OR EVEN TRACK YOUR SUPPS AND MACROS.

DATE		DAY		TIME		WT	
MOOD				ENERGY LEVEL		1 2 3 4 5	
PROGRAM				PARTNER			

MUSCLE FOCUS				LOCATION				
STRENGTH TRAINING	S1	S2	S3	S4	S5	SET TYPE	EQUIP-MENT	P.R.

CALS BURNED	END TIME		DURATION	
CARDIO	DURATION	DISTANCE		INTENSITY

CALS BURNED	SUPPS USED	
HOW WAS MY WORKOUT?	1 2 3 4 5 6 7 8 9 10	

HYDRATE!

| 1 | = 8 OZ |

AIM TO CHECK OFF ALL 16 BOXES, ESPECIALLY ON WORKOUT DAYS.

2	3	4	5	6
7	8	9	10	11
12	13	14	15	16

FIT TIP:
Willpower is not a talent; it is a muscle that is developed by *using* it.

WHAT AM I DOING WELL?

QUOTE OF THE DAY:
Never, never, never give up.
        - Sir Winston Churchill

HOW CAN I IMPROVE?

WHO CAN I ENCOURAGE OR PRAY FOR TODAY?

1.

MY COMMITMENT TO MYSELF TODAY:

2.

3.

LET IT ALL OUT!

WRITE YOUR FOOD STRUGGLES, MOTIVATION ISSUES, OR EVEN TRACK YOUR SUPPS AND MACROS.

DATE		DAY		TIME		WT	
MOOD				ENERGY LEVEL		1 2 3 4 5	
PROGRAM				PARTNER			

MUSCLE FOCUS / LOCATION

STRENGTH TRAINING	S1	S2	S3	S4	S5	SET TYPE	EQUIP-MENT	P.R.

CALS BURNED	END TIME		DURATION	
CARDIO	DURATION	DISTANCE	INTENSITY	

CALS BURNED	SUPPS USED	
HOW WAS MY WORKOUT?	1 2 3 4 5 6 7 8 9 10	

HYDRATE!

AIM TO CHECK OFF ALL 16 BOXES, ESPECIALLY ON WORKOUT DAYS.

1	= 8 OZ			
2	3	4	5	6
7	8	9	10	11
12	13	14	15	16

FIT TIP:
Make a fitness wish list, and each time you meet a goal, reward yourself with something from your list.

WHAT AM I DOING WELL?

QUOTE OF THE DAY:
You may be disappointed if you fail, but you are doomed if you don't try.
— Beverly Sills

HOW CAN I IMPROVE?

WHO CAN I ENCOURAGE OR PRAY FOR TODAY?

1.

2.

MY COMMITMENT TO MYSELF TODAY:

3.

LET IT ALL OUT!

WRITE YOUR FOOD STRUGGLES, MOTIVATION ISSUES, OR EVEN TRACK YOUR SUPPS AND MACROS.

DATE		DAY		TIME		WT	
MOOD				ENERGY LEVEL		1 2 3 4 5	
PROGRAM				PARTNER			

MUSCLE FOCUS				LOCATION				
STRENGTH TRAINING	S1	S2	S3	S4	S5	SET TYPE	EQUIP-MENT	P.R.

CALS BURNED	END TIME		DURATION	
CARDIO	DURATION	DISTANCE		INTENSITY

CALS BURNED	SUPPS USED	
HOW WAS MY WORKOUT?	1 2 3 4 5 6 7 8 9 10	

HYDRATE!

AIM TO CHECK OFF ALL 16 BOXES, ESPECIALLY ON WORKOUT DAYS.

1	= 8 OZ			
2	3	4	5	6
7	8	9	10	11
12	13	14	15	16

FIT TIP:
If you restrict too much, there is an increased risk of a binge, which can lead to more poor decisions and cause a major setback.

WHAT AM I DOING WELL?

QUOTE OF THE DAY:
There is no substitute for hard work.
- Thomas Edison

HOW CAN I IMPROVE?

WHO CAN I ENCOURAGE OR PRAY FOR TODAY?

1.

MY COMMITMENT TO MYSELF TODAY:

2.

3.

LET IT ALL OUT!

WRITE YOUR FOOD STRUGGLES, MOTIVATION ISSUES, OR EVEN TRACK YOUR SUPPS AND MACROS.

IF YOU FAIL TO PLAN...

GOALS FOR THIS WEEK
Specific | **M**easurable | **A**ttainable | **R**ealistic | **T**ime-Bound

Example: I will drink one gallon of water each day this week.

1.

2.

3.

POTIENTIAL ROADBLOCKS	VECTOR CHECK
Anticipate what might throw you off track and plan a solution.	Check each of your written goals and evaluate your progress.
HAZARD: Business luncheon Thurs.	Are you on track to meet your goal?
DETOUR: Protein shake before lunch	
HAZARD:	
	If not, why?
DETOUR:	
HAZARD:	What can you do to get back on track?
DETOUR	
	If you need to modify your goals, do it now!

...YOU ARE PLANNING TO FAIL.

— Benjamin Franklin

MEAL PLANNING
Plan a menu - OR - Write down your meals - OR - Make a grocery list.

SUNDAY

MONDAY

TUESDAY

WEDNESDAY

THURSDAY

FRIDAY
Caution: weekend ahead!

SATURDAY

EXAMPLE A

- M1 - oats, protein shake
- M2 - whole grain toast & cheese
- M3 - scrambled egg white sandwich w/spinach
- M4 - carrots & hummus
- M5 - chicken, rice, veggies
- M6 - pizza (oops!)

EXAMPLE B

- Make turkey chili and protein bars
- Go grocery shopping
- Date Night! Look up restaurant menu

DATE		DAY		TIME		WT	
MOOD				ENERGY LEVEL		1 2 3 4 5	
PROGRAM				PARTNER			

MUSCLE FOCUS				LOCATION				
STRENGTH TRAINING	S1	S2	S3	S4	S5	SET TYPE	EQUIP-MENT	P.R.

CALS BURNED	END TIME		DURATION	
CARDIO	DURATION	DISTANCE		INTENSITY

CALS BURNED	SUPPS USED	
HOW WAS MY WORKOUT?	1 2 3 4 5	6 7 8 9 10

HYDRATE!

AIM TO CHECK OFF ALL 16 BOXES, ESPECIALLY ON WORKOUT DAYS.

1	= 8 OZ			
2	3	4	5	6
7	8	9	10	11
12	13	14	15	16

FIT TIP:
For fat loss, try fasted cardio first thing in the morning.

WHAT AM I DOING WELL?

QUOTE OF THE DAY:
Do what you can, with what you have, where you are.
— Theodore Roosevelt

HOW CAN I IMPROVE?

WHO CAN I ENCOURAGE OR PRAY FOR TODAY?

1.

MY COMMITMENT TO MYSELF TODAY:

2.

3.

LET IT ALL OUT!

WRITE YOUR FOOD STRUGGLES, MOTIVATION ISSUES, OR EVEN TRACK YOUR SUPPS AND MACROS.

DATE		DAY		TIME		WT	
MOOD				ENERGY LEVEL		1 2 3 4 5	
PROGRAM				PARTNER			

MUSCLE FOCUS				LOCATION				
STRENGTH TRAINING	S1	S2	S3	S4	S5	SET TYPE	EQUIPMENT	P.R.

CALS BURNED	END TIME		DURATION	
CARDIO	DURATION	DISTANCE		INTENSITY

CALS BURNED	SUPPS USED	
HOW WAS MY WORKOUT?		1 2 3 4 5 6 7 8 9 10

HYDRATE!

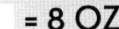 = 8 OZ

AIM TO CHECK OFF ALL 16 BOXES, ESPECIALLY ON WORKOUT DAYS.

2	3	4	5	6
7	8	9	10	11
12	13	14	15	16

FIT TIP:
Make a plan, then give it time to work. People often fail just because they quit too soon.

WHAT AM I DOING WELL?

QUOTE OF THE DAY:
Be strong and courageous.
— Joshua 1:9

HOW CAN I IMPROVE?

WHO CAN I ENCOURAGE OR PRAY FOR TODAY?

1.

MY COMMITMENT TO MYSELF TODAY:

2.

3.

LET IT ALL OUT!

WRITE YOUR FOOD STRUGGLES, MOTIVATION ISSUES, OR EVEN TRACK YOUR SUPPS AND MACROS.

DATE		DAY		TIME		WT	
MOOD				ENERGY LEVEL		**1** 2 3 4 5	
PROGRAM				PARTNER			

MUSCLE FOCUS				LOCATION					
STRENGTH TRAINING	S1	S2	S3	S4	S5	SET TYPE	EQUIP-MENT	P.R.	

CALS BURNED	END TIME		DURATION	
CARDIO	DURATION	DISTANCE		INTENSITY

CALS BURNED	SUPPS USED	
HOW WAS MY WORKOUT?	**1** 2 3 4 5 6 7 8 9 10	

HYDRATE!

AIM TO CHECK OFF ALL 16 BOXES, ESPECIALLY ON WORKOUT DAYS.

1	2	3	4	5	6
7	8	9	10	11	
12	13	14	15	16	

= 8 OZ

FIT TIP:
If you hit a plateau, it is more likely that your diet is to blame than your workouts.

WHAT AM I DOING WELL?

QUOTE OF THE DAY:
I attribute my success to this:
I never gave or took an excuse.
— Florence Nightingale

HOW CAN I IMPROVE?

WHO CAN I ENCOURAGE OR PRAY FOR TODAY?

1.

MY COMMITMENT TO MYSELF TODAY:

2.

3.

LET IT ALL OUT!

WRITE YOUR FOOD STRUGGLES, MOTIVATION ISSUES, OR EVEN TRACK YOUR SUPPS AND MACROS.

DATE		DAY		TIME		WT	
MOOD				ENERGY LEVEL		1 2 3 4 5	
PROGRAM				PARTNER			

MUSCLE FOCUS				LOCATION				
STRENGTH TRAINING	S1	S2	S3	S4	S5	SET TYPE	EQUIPMENT	P.R.

CALS BURNED	END TIME		DURATION	
CARDIO	DURATION	DISTANCE		INTENSITY

CALS BURNED	SUPPS USED	
HOW WAS MY WORKOUT?		1 2 3 4 5 6 7 8 9 10

HYDRATE!

☐ = 8 OZ

AIM TO CHECK OFF ALL 16 BOXES, ESPECIALLY ON WORKOUT DAYS.

1	2	3	4	5	6
	7	8	9	10	11
	12	13	14	15	16

FIT TIP:
Consider flexible dieting, or IIFYM. It allows flexibility in your food choices and is a game changer for many.

WHAT AM I DOING WELL?

QUOTE OF THE DAY:
We learn to walk by stumbling.
— Bulgarian proverb

HOW CAN I IMPROVE?

WHO CAN I ENCOURAGE OR PRAY FOR TODAY?

1.

MY COMMITMENT TO MYSELF TODAY:

2.

3.

LET IT ALL OUT!

WRITE YOUR FOOD STRUGGLES, MOTIVATION ISSUES, OR EVEN TRACK YOUR SUPPS AND MACROS.

DATE		DAY		TIME		WT	
MOOD				ENERGY LEVEL		1 2 3 4 5	
PROGRAM				PARTNER			

MUSCLE FOCUS				LOCATION				
STRENGTH TRAINING	S1	S2	S3	S4	S5	SET TYPE	EQUIPMENT	P.R.

CALS BURNED	END TIME		DURATION	
CARDIO	DURATION	DISTANCE		INTENSITY

CALS BURNED	SUPPS USED	
HOW WAS MY WORKOUT?		1 2 3 4 5 6 7 8 9 10

HYDRATE!

AIM TO CHECK OFF ALL 16 BOXES, ESPECIALLY ON WORKOUT DAYS.

1	= 8 OZ			
2	3	4	5	6
7	8	9	10	11
12	13	14	15	16

FIT TIP:
If you change everything at once, you're setting yourself up for failure. Make small, sustainable changes over time to set yourself up for long-term success!

WHAT AM I DOING WELL?

QUOTE OF THE DAY:
Sometimes the best helping hand you can get is a good, firm push.
— Joann Thomas

HOW CAN I IMPROVE?

WHO CAN I ENCOURAGE OR PRAY FOR TODAY?

1.

MY COMMITMENT TO MYSELF TODAY:

2.

3.

LET IT ALL OUT!

WRITE YOUR FOOD STRUGGLES, MOTIVATION ISSUES, OR EVEN TRACK YOUR SUPPS AND MACROS.

DATE		DAY		TIME		WT	
MOOD				ENERGY LEVEL		1 2 3 4 5	
PROGRAM				PARTNER			

MUSCLE FOCUS				LOCATION				
STRENGTH TRAINING	S1	S2	S3	S4	S5	SET TYPE	EQUIP-MENT	P.R.

CALS BURNED	END TIME		DURATION	
CARDIO	DURATION	DISTANCE		INTENSITY

CALS BURNED	SUPPS USED	
HOW WAS MY WORKOUT?	1 2 3 4 5 6 7 8 9 10	

HYDRATE!

1 = 8 OZ

AIM TO CHECK OFF ALL 16 BOXES, ESPECIALLY ON WORKOUT DAYS.

2	3	4	5	6
7	8	9	10	11
12	13	14	15	16

FIT TIP:
Find a partner, set up a schedule of sharing progress photos every 3-4 weeks, and provide honest feedback, with the agreement there are no hurt feelings.

WHAT AM I DOING WELL?

QUOTE OF THE DAY:
When the world says, 'Give up;' Hope whispers, 'Try it one more time.'
– Author unknown

HOW CAN I IMPROVE?

WHO CAN I ENCOURAGE OR PRAY FOR TODAY?

1.

MY COMMITMENT TO MYSELF TODAY:

2.

3.

LET IT ALL OUT!

WRITE YOUR FOOD STRUGGLES, MOTIVATION ISSUES, OR EVEN TRACK YOUR SUPPS AND MACROS.

DATE _____ DAY _____ TIME _____ WT _____
MOOD _____ ENERGY LEVEL **1** 2 3 4 5
PROGRAM _____ PARTNER _____

MUSCLE FOCUS	LOCATION							
STRENGTH TRAINING	S1	S2	S3	S4	S5	SET TYPE	EQUIP-MENT	P.R.

CALS BURNED	END TIME	DURATION
CARDIO	DURATION	DISTANCE	INTENSITY

CALS BURNED	SUPPS USED
HOW WAS MY WORKOUT?	**1** 2 3 4 5 6 7 8 9 10

HYDRATE!

☐ = 8 OZ

AIM TO CHECK OFF ALL 16 BOXES, ESPECIALLY ON WORKOUT DAYS.

1	2	3	4	5	6
7	8	9	10	11
12	13	14	15	16

FIT TIP:
Life happens. Things will not always go smoothly or as planned. When that happens, make adjustments and keep going.

WHAT AM I DOING WELL?

QUOTE OF THE DAY:
Refuse to be average. Let your heart soar as high as it will.
— A.W. Tozer

HOW CAN I IMPROVE?

WHO CAN I ENCOURAGE OR PRAY FOR TODAY?

1.

MY COMMITMENT TO MYSELF TODAY:

2.

3.

LET IT ALL OUT!

WRITE YOUR FOOD STRUGGLES, MOTIVATION ISSUES, OR EVEN TRACK YOUR SUPPS AND MACROS.

IF YOU FAIL TO PLAN...

GOALS FOR THIS WEEK
Specific | **M**easurable | **A**ttainable | **R**ealistic | **T**ime-Bound

Example: I will drink one gallon of water each day this week.

1.

2.

3.

POTIENTIAL ROADBLOCKS	VECTOR CHECK
Anticipate what might throw you off track and plan a solution.	Check each of your written goals and evaluate your progress.
HAZARD: Business luncheon Thurs.	Are you on track to meet your goal?
DETOUR: Protein shake before lunch	
HAZARD:	
	If not, why?
DETOUR:	
HAZARD:	What can you do to get back on track?
DETOUR	
	If you need to modify your goals, do it now!

...YOU ARE PLANNING TO FAIL.

— Benjamin Franklin

MEAL PLANNING
Plan a menu - OR - Write down your meals - OR - Make a grocery list.

SUNDAY

MONDAY

TUESDAY

WEDNESDAY

THURSDAY

FRIDAY
Caution: weekend ahead!

SATURDAY

EXAMPLE A

M1 - oats, protein shake
M2 - whole grain toast & cheese
M3 - scrambled egg white sandwich w/spinach
M4 - carrots & hummus
M5 - chicken, rice, veggies
M6 - pizza (oops!)

EXAMPLE B

- Make turkey chili and protein bars

- Go grocery shopping

- Date Night! Look up restaurant menu

DATE		DAY		TIME		WT	
MOOD				ENERGY LEVEL		1 2 3 4 5	
PROGRAM				PARTNER			

MUSCLE FOCUS				LOCATION				
STRENGTH TRAINING	S1	S2	S3	S4	S5	SET TYPE	EQUIP-MENT	P.R.

CALS BURNED	END TIME		DURATION	
CARDIO	DURATION	DISTANCE		INTENSITY

CALS BURNED	SUPPS USED	
HOW WAS MY WORKOUT?	1 2 3 4 5 6 7 8 9 10	

HYDRATE!

AIM TO CHECK OFF ALL 16 BOXES, ESPECIALLY ON WORKOUT DAYS.

[1] = 8 OZ

2	3	4	5	6
7	8	9	10	11
12	13	14	15	16

FIT TIP:
You can achieve your fitness goals without spending hours in the gym each day. Intensity and consistency are important.

WHAT AM I DOING WELL?

QUOTE OF THE DAY:
Learn from yesterday, live for today, hope for tomorrow.
— Albert Einstein

HOW CAN I IMPROVE?

WHO CAN I ENCOURAGE OR PRAY FOR TODAY?

1.

MY COMMITMENT TO MYSELF TODAY:

2.

3.

LET IT ALL OUT!

WRITE YOUR FOOD STRUGGLES, MOTIVATION ISSUES, OR EVEN TRACK YOUR SUPPS AND MACROS.

DATE		DAY		TIME		WT	
MOOD				ENERGY LEVEL		1 2 3 4 5	
PROGRAM				PARTNER			

MUSCLE FOCUS				LOCATION					
STRENGTH TRAINING	S1	S2	S3	S4	S5	SET TYPE	EQUIP-MENT	P.R.

CALS BURNED	END TIME		DURATION	
CARDIO	DURATION	DISTANCE	INTENSITY	

CALS BURNED	SUPPS USED	
HOW WAS MY WORKOUT?	1 2 3 4 5 6 7 8 9 10	

HYDRATE!

AIM TO CHECK OFF ALL 16 BOXES, ESPECIALLY ON WORKOUT DAYS.

1	= 8 OZ

2	3	4	5	6
7	8	9	10	11
12	13	14	15	16

FIT TIP:
Log your workouts *and* your food intake. You can't figure out where you need to go if you don't know where you've been.

WHAT AM I DOING WELL?

QUOTE OF THE DAY:
The future depends on what we do in the present.
— Mahatma Gandhi

HOW CAN I IMPROVE?

WHO CAN I ENCOURAGE OR PRAY FOR TODAY?

1.

MY COMMITMENT TO MYSELF TODAY:

2.

3.

LET IT ALL OUT!

WRITE YOUR FOOD STRUGGLES, MOTIVATION ISSUES, OR EVEN TRACK YOUR SUPPS AND MACROS.

DATE		DAY		TIME		WT	
MOOD			ENERGY LEVEL		1 2 3 4 5		
PROGRAM			PARTNER				

MUSCLE FOCUS				LOCATION				
STRENGTH TRAINING	S1	S2	S3	S4	S5	SET TYPE	EQUIP-MENT	P.R.

CALS BURNED	END TIME		DURATION	
CARDIO	DURATION	DISTANCE		INTENSITY

CALS BURNED	SUPPS USED	
HOW WAS MY WORKOUT?	1 2 3 4 5 6 7 8 9 10	

HYDRATE!

AIM TO CHECK OFF ALL 16 BOXES, ESPECIALLY ON WORKOUT DAYS.

| 1 | = 8 OZ |

2	3	4	5	6
7	8	9	10	11
12	13	14	15	16

FIT TIP:
Many factors affect the scale: water retention, hormones, and sodium intake, to name a few. An increase on the scale may not indicate fat gain.

WHAT AM I DOING WELL?

QUOTE OF THE DAY:
There is nothing entirely within our power but our own thoughts.
— Rene Descartes

HOW CAN I IMPROVE?

WHO CAN I ENCOURAGE OR PRAY FOR TODAY?

1.

MY COMMITMENT TO MYSELF TODAY:

2.

3.

LET IT ALL OUT!

WRITE YOUR FOOD STRUGGLES, MOTIVATION ISSUES, OR EVEN TRACK YOUR SUPPS AND MACROS.

DATE		DAY		TIME		WT	
MOOD				ENERGY LEVEL		**1** 2 3 4 5	
PROGRAM				PARTNER			

MUSCLE FOCUS					LOCATION			
STRENGTH TRAINING	S1	S2	S3	S4	S5	SET TYPE	EQUIP-MENT	P.R.

CALS BURNED	END TIME		DURATION	
CARDIO	DURATION	DISTANCE		INTENSITY

CALS BURNED	SUPPS USED	
HOW WAS MY WORKOUT?	1 2 3 4 5 6 7 8 9 10	

HYDRATE!

| 1 | = 8 OZ |

AIM TO CHECK OFF ALL 16 BOXES, ESPECIALLY ON WORKOUT DAYS.

2	3	4	5	6
7	8	9	10	11
12	13	14	15	16

FIT TIP:
Hydrate! Water is not only important just for overall health, but it keeps your metabolism running efficiently.

WHAT AM I DOING WELL?

QUOTE OF THE DAY:
The greater the obstacle, the more glory in overcoming it.
— Jean-Baptist Molière

HOW CAN I IMPROVE?

WHO CAN I ENCOURAGE OR PRAY FOR TODAY?

1.

MY COMMITMENT TO MYSELF TODAY:

2.

3.

LET IT ALL OUT!

WRITE YOUR FOOD STRUGGLES, MOTIVATION ISSUES, OR EVEN TRACK YOUR SUPPS AND MACROS.

DATE		DAY		TIME		WT	

MOOD ENERGY LEVEL **1 2 3 4 5**

PROGRAM PARTNER

MUSCLE FOCUS / LOCATION

STRENGTH TRAINING	S1	S2	S3	S4	S5	SET TYPE	EQUIP-MENT	P.R.

CALS BURNED END TIME DURATION

CARDIO	DURATION	DISTANCE	INTENSITY

CALS BURNED SUPPS USED

HOW WAS MY WORKOUT? **1 2 3 4 5 6 7 8 9 10**

HYDRATE!

AIM TO CHECK OFF ALL 16 BOXES, ESPECIALLY ON WORKOUT DAYS.

[1] = 8 OZ

2	3	4	5	6
7	8	9	10	11
12	13	14	15	16

FIT TIP:
Consider supplements. They can be intimidating, but adding a few supplements can help you reach your goals faster.

WHAT AM I DOING WELL?

QUOTE OF THE DAY:
When you want to succeed as bad as you want to breathe, then you will be successful.
— Eric Thomas

HOW CAN I IMPROVE?

WHO CAN I ENCOURAGE OR PRAY FOR TODAY?

1.

MY COMMITMENT TO MYSELF TODAY:

2.

3.

LET IT ALL OUT!

WRITE YOUR FOOD STRUGGLES, MOTIVATION ISSUES, OR EVEN TRACK YOUR SUPPS AND MACROS.

DATE		DAY		TIME		WT	

MOOD ENERGY LEVEL 1 2 3 4 5
PROGRAM PARTNER

MUSCLE FOCUS / LOCATION

STRENGTH TRAINING	S1	S2	S3	S4	S5	SET TYPE	EQUIP-MENT	P.R.

CALS BURNED	END TIME		DURATION	
CARDIO	DURATION	DISTANCE		INTENSITY

CALS BURNED	SUPPS USED	
HOW WAS MY WORKOUT?	1 2 3 4 5 6 7 8 9 10	

HYDRATE!

☐ = 8 OZ

AIM TO CHECK OFF ALL 16 BOXES, ESPECIALLY ON WORKOUT DAYS.

2	3	4	5	6
7	8	9	10	11
12	13	14	15	16

FIT TIP:
When heading to a social event, eat or have a protein shake before you go. It'll be easier to ignore the dessert table if you aren't famished.

WHAT AM I DOING WELL?

QUOTE OF THE DAY:
I press on toward the goal to win the prize for which God has called me heavenward in Christ Jesus.
 - Philippians 3:14

HOW CAN I IMPROVE?

WHO CAN I ENCOURAGE OR PRAY FOR TODAY?

1.

MY COMMITMENT TO MYSELF TODAY:

2.

3.

LET IT ALL OUT!

WRITE YOUR FOOD STRUGGLES, MOTIVATION ISSUES, OR EVEN TRACK YOUR SUPPS AND MACROS.

DATE		DAY		TIME		WT	
MOOD			ENERGY LEVEL		1 2 3 4 5		
PROGRAM			PARTNER				

MUSCLE FOCUS			LOCATION					
STRENGTH TRAINING	S1	S2	S3	S4	S5	SET TYPE	EQUIP-MENT	P.R.

CALS BURNED	END TIME		DURATION	
CARDIO	DURATION	DISTANCE		INTENSITY

CALS BURNED	SUPPS USED	
HOW WAS MY WORKOUT?	1 2 3 4 5 6 7 8 9 10	

HYDRATE!

□ = 8 OZ

AIM TO CHECK OFF ALL 16 BOXES, ESPECIALLY ON WORKOUT DAYS.

2	3	4	5	6
7	8	9	10	11
12	13	14	15	16

FIT TIP:
Take measurements. Bust, waist, hips and thighs especially. Take them monthly, at the same time of day, and compare your progress!

WHAT AM I DOING WELL?

QUOTE OF THE DAY:
Action will destroy your procrastination.
— Og Mandino

HOW CAN I IMPROVE?

WHO CAN I ENCOURAGE OR PRAY FOR TODAY?

1.

MY COMMITMENT TO MYSELF TODAY:

2.

3.

LET IT ALL OUT!

WRITE YOUR FOOD STRUGGLES, MOTIVATION ISSUES, OR EVEN TRACK YOUR SUPPS AND MACROS.

IF YOU FAIL TO PLAN...

GOALS FOR THIS WEEK
Specific | **M**easurable | **A**ttainable | **R**ealistic | **T**ime-Bound

Example: I will drink one gallon of water each day this week.

1.

2.

3.

POTIENTIAL ROADBLOCKS	VECTOR CHECK
Anticipate what might throw you off track and plan a solution.	Check each of your written goals and evaluate your progress.
HAZARD: Business luncheon Thurs.	Are you on track to meet your goal?
DETOUR: Protein shake before lunch	
HAZARD:	
	If not, why?
DETOUR:	
HAZARD:	What can you do to get back on track?
DETOUR	
	If you need to modify your goals, do it now!

...YOU ARE PLANNING TO FAIL.

— Benjamin Franklin

MEAL PLANNING
Plan a menu - OR - Write down your meals - OR - Make a grocery list.

SUNDAY

MONDAY

TUESDAY

WEDNESDAY

THURSDAY

FRIDAY
Caution: weekend ahead!

SATURDAY

EXAMPLE A

- M1 – oats, protein shake
- M2 – whole grain toast & cheese
- M3 – scrambled egg white sandwich w/spinach
- M4 – carrots & hummus
- M5 – chicken, rice, veggies
- M6 – pizza (oops!)

EXAMPLE B

- Make turkey chili and protein bars
- Go grocery shopping
- Date Night! Look up restaurant menu

DATE		DAY		TIME		WT	
MOOD				ENERGY LEVEL		1 2 3 4 5	
PROGRAM				PARTNER			

MUSCLE FOCUS				LOCATION				
STRENGTH TRAINING	S1	S2	S3	S4	S5	SET TYPE	EQUIP-MENT	P.R.

CALS BURNED	END TIME		DURATION	
CARDIO	DURATION	DISTANCE		INTENSITY

CALS BURNED	SUPPS USED	
HOW WAS MY WORKOUT?	1 2 3 4 5 6 7 8 9 10	

HYDRATE!

☐ = 8 OZ

AIM TO CHECK OFF ALL 16 BOXES, ESPECIALLY ON WORKOUT DAYS.

2	3	4	5	6
7	8	9	10	11
12	13	14	15	16

FIT TIP:
Carry around a water bottle. It's difficult to stay sufficiently hydrated if you aren't intentional about your intake.

WHAT AM I DOING WELL?

QUOTE OF THE DAY:
Spectacular achievement is always preceded by spectacular preparation.
  - Robert H. Schuller

HOW CAN I IMPROVE?

WHO CAN I ENCOURAGE OR PRAY FOR TODAY?

1.

MY COMMITMENT TO MYSELF TODAY:

2.

3.

LET IT ALL OUT!

WRITE YOUR FOOD STRUGGLES, MOTIVATION ISSUES, OR EVEN TRACK YOUR SUPPS AND MACROS.

DATE		DAY		TIME		WT	
MOOD				ENERGY LEVEL		1 2 3 4 5	
PROGRAM				PARTNER			

MUSCLE FOCUS				LOCATION					
STRENGTH TRAINING	S1	S2	S3	S4	S5	SET TYPE	EQUIP-MENT	P.R.

CALS BURNED	END TIME		DURATION	
CARDIO	DURATION	DISTANCE		INTENSITY

CALS BURNED	SUPPS USED	
HOW WAS MY WORKOUT?	1 2 3 4 5 6 7 8 9 10	

HYDRATE!

AIM TO CHECK OFF ALL 16 BOXES, ESPECIALLY ON WORKOUT DAYS.

☐ 1 = 8 OZ

2	3	4	5	6
7	8	9	10	11
12	13	14	15	16

FIT TIP:
If you find it difficult to wake up for your workouts, set your alarm clock across the room so you have to get up to turn it off.

WHAT AM I DOING WELL?

QUOTE OF THE DAY:
When you are through changing, you are through.
— Bruce Barton

HOW CAN I IMPROVE?

WHO CAN I ENCOURAGE OR PRAY FOR TODAY?

1.

MY COMMITMENT TO MYSELF TODAY:

2.

3.

LET IT ALL OUT!

WRITE YOUR FOOD STRUGGLES, MOTIVATION ISSUES, OR EVEN TRACK YOUR SUPPS AND MACROS.

DATE		DAY		TIME		WT	

MOOD   ENERGY LEVEL   **1** 2 3 4 5

PROGRAM   PARTNER

MUSCLE FOCUS   LOCATION

STRENGTH TRAINING	S1	S2	S3	S4	S5	SET TYPE	EQUIP-MENT	P.R.

CALS BURNED   END TIME   DURATION

CARDIO	DURATION	DISTANCE	INTENSITY

CALS BURNED   SUPPS USED

HOW WAS MY WORKOUT?   1   2   3   4   5   6   7   8   9   10

HYDRATE!

☐ = 8 OZ

AIM TO CHECK OFF ALL 16 BOXES, ESPECIALLY ON WORKOUT DAYS.

1	2	3	4	5	6
7	8	9	10	11
12	13	14	15	16

FIT TIP:

Get some sleep. Lack of rest impedes fat loss. Know your body and get the amount of sleep it needs. If necessary, take an afternoon power nap!

WHAT AM I DOING WELL?

QUOTE OF THE DAY:

Success is the sum of small efforts, repeated day in and day out.
— Robert Collier

HOW CAN I IMPROVE?

WHO CAN I ENCOURAGE OR PRAY FOR TODAY?

1.

MY COMMITMENT TO MYSELF TODAY:

2.

3.

LET IT ALL OUT!

WRITE YOUR FOOD STRUGGLES, MOTIVATION ISSUES, OR EVEN TRACK YOUR SUPPS AND MACROS.

DATE　　　　　　DAY　　　　　　TIME　　　　　　WT
MOOD　　　　　　　　　ENERGY LEVEL　　1 2 3 4 5
PROGRAM　　　　　　　　　　PARTNER

MUSCLE FOCUS			LOCATION					
STRENGTH TRAINING	S1	S2	S3	S4	S5	SET TYPE	EQUIP-MENT	P.R.

CALS BURNED	END TIME		DURATION	
CARDIO	DURATION	DISTANCE		INTENSITY

CALS BURNED	SUPPS USED									
HOW WAS MY WORKOUT?	1	2	3	4	5	6	7	8	9	10

HYDRATE!

☐ = 8 OZ

AIM TO CHECK OFF ALL 16 BOXES, ESPECIALLY ON WORKOUT DAYS.

1	2	3	4	5	6
	7	8	9	10	11
	12	13	14	15	16

FIT TIP:
You can bank calories for a special occasion. Drop your calories slightly through the week to save up for the feast on your special day!

WHAT AM I DOING WELL?

QUOTE OF THE DAY:
What is necessary to change a person is to change his awareness of himself.
— Abraham Maslow

HOW CAN I IMPROVE?

WHO CAN I ENCOURAGE OR PRAY FOR TODAY?

1.

MY COMMITMENT TO MYSELF TODAY:

2.

3.

LET IT ALL OUT!

WRITE YOUR FOOD STRUGGLES, MOTIVATION ISSUES, OR EVEN TRACK YOUR SUPPS AND MACROS.

DATE		DAY		TIME		WT	
MOOD			ENERGY LEVEL		1 2 3 4 5		
PROGRAM				PARTNER			

MUSCLE FOCUS				LOCATION				
STRENGTH TRAINING	S1	S2	S3	S4	S5	SET TYPE	EQUIP-MENT	P.R.

CALS BURNED	END TIME		DURATION	
CARDIO	DURATION	DISTANCE	INTENSITY	

CALS BURNED	SUPPS USED	
HOW WAS MY WORKOUT?	1 2 3 4 5 6 7 8 9 10	

HYDRATE!

1 = 8 OZ

AIM TO CHECK OFF ALL 16 BOXES, ESPECIALLY ON WORKOUT DAYS.

2	3	4	5	6
7	8	9	10	11
12	13	14	15	16

FIT TIP:
If you struggle to find time to exercise, keep a time log. You'll be surprised how much extra time you find when you are intentional with how you spend it!

WHAT AM I DOING WELL?

QUOTE OF THE DAY:
The important thing is not to stop questioning. Curiosity has its own reason for existing.

— Albert Einstein

HOW CAN I IMPROVE?

WHO CAN I ENCOURAGE OR PRAY FOR TODAY?

1.

MY COMMITMENT TO MYSELF TODAY:

2.

3.

LET IT ALL OUT!

WRITE YOUR FOOD STRUGGLES, MOTIVATION ISSUES, OR EVEN TRACK YOUR SUPPS AND MACROS.

DATE		DAY		TIME		WT	
MOOD				ENERGY LEVEL		1 2 3 4 5	
PROGRAM				PARTNER			

MUSCLE FOCUS / LOCATION

STRENGTH TRAINING	S1	S2	S3	S4	S5	SET TYPE	EQUIP-MENT	P.R.

CALS BURNED	END TIME		DURATION	
CARDIO	DURATION	DISTANCE		INTENSITY

CALS BURNED	SUPPS USED	
HOW WAS MY WORKOUT?	1 2 3 4 5 6 7 8 9 10	

HYDRATE!

1 = 8 OZ

AIM TO CHECK OFF ALL 16 BOXES, ESPECIALLY ON WORKOUT DAYS.

1	2	3	4	5	6
7	8	9	10	11	
12	13	14	15	16	

FIT TIP:
Each week, take a few moments to think through the next seven days. Anticipate roadblocks and opportunities to excel. Only you can ensure a successful week.

WHAT AM I DOING WELL?

QUOTE OF THE DAY:
Whatever the mind can conceive and believe, the mind can achieve.
— Napoleon Hill.

HOW CAN I IMPROVE?

WHO CAN I ENCOURAGE OR PRAY FOR TODAY?

1.

MY COMMITMENT TO MYSELF TODAY:

2.

3.

LET IT ALL OUT!

WRITE YOUR FOOD STRUGGLES, MOTIVATION ISSUES, OR EVEN TRACK YOUR SUPPS AND MACROS.

DATE		DAY		TIME		WT	
MOOD				ENERGY LEVEL		1 2 3 4 5	
PROGRAM				PARTNER			

MUSCLE FOCUS				LOCATION				
STRENGTH TRAINING	S1	S2	S3	S4	S5	SET TYPE	EQUIP-MENT	P.R.

CALS BURNED	END TIME		DURATION	
CARDIO	DURATION	DISTANCE		INTENSITY

CALS BURNED	SUPPS USED	
HOW WAS MY WORKOUT?	1 2 3 4 5 6 7 8 9 10	

HYDRATE!

1 = 8 OZ

AIM TO CHECK OFF ALL 16 BOXES, ESPECIALLY ON WORKOUT DAYS.

1	2	3	4	5	6
	7	8	9	10	11
	12	13	14	15	16

FIT TIP:
Teach others how to treat you. If others try to sabotage your success, you must communicate to them that is not acceptable.

WHAT AM I DOING WELL?

QUOTE OF THE DAY:
Even if you are on the right track, you'll get run over if you just sit there.
— Will Rogers

HOW CAN I IMPROVE?

WHO CAN I ENCOURAGE OR PRAY FOR TODAY?

1.

MY COMMITMENT TO MYSELF TODAY:

2.

3.

LET IT ALL OUT!

WRITE YOUR FOOD STRUGGLES, MOTIVATION ISSUES, OR EVEN TRACK YOUR SUPPS AND MACROS.

IF YOU FAIL TO PLAN...

GOALS FOR THIS WEEK
Specific | **M**easurable | **A**ttainable | **R**ealistic | **T**ime-Bound

Example: I will drink one gallon of water each day this week.

1.

2.

3.

POTIENTIAL ROADBLOCKS

Anticipate what might throw you off track and plan a solution.

HAZARD: Business luncheon Thurs.

DETOUR: Protein shake before lunch

HAZARD:

DETOUR:

HAZARD:

DETOUR

VECTOR CHECK

Check each of your written goals and evaluate your progress.

Are you on track to meet your goal?

If not, why?

What can you do to get back on track?

If you need to modify your goals, do it now!

...YOU ARE PLANNING TO FAIL.

— Benjamin Franklin

MEAL PLANNING
Plan a menu - OR - Write down your meals - OR - Make a grocery list.

SUNDAY

MONDAY

TUESDAY

WEDNESDAY

THURSDAY

FRIDAY
Caution: weekend ahead!

SATURDAY

EXAMPLE A

- M1 - oats, protein shake
- M2 - whole grain toast & cheese
- M3 - scrambled egg white sandwich w/spinach
- M4 - carrots & hummus
- M5 - chicken, rice, veggies
- M6 - pizza (oops!)

EXAMPLE B

- Make turkey chili and protein bars
- Go grocery shopping
- Date Night! Look up restaurant menu

DATE		DAY		TIME		WT	
MOOD				ENERGY LEVEL		1 2 3 4 5	
PROGRAM				PARTNER			

MUSCLE FOCUS				LOCATION			
STRENGTH TRAINING	S1	S2	S3	S4	S5	SET TYPE	EQUIPMENT	P.R.

CALS BURNED	END TIME		DURATION	
CARDIO	DURATION	DISTANCE		INTENSITY

CALS BURNED	SUPPS USED	
HOW WAS MY WORKOUT?	1 2 3 4 5 6 7 8 9 10	

HYDRATE!

AIM TO CHECK OFF ALL 16 BOXES, ESPECIALLY ON WORKOUT DAYS.

1					= 8 OZ

2	3	4	5	6
7	8	9	10	11
12	13	14	15	16

FIT TIP:
Be honest with yourself, know your limitations, and set yourself up for success with decisions you make.

WHAT AM I DOING WELL?

QUOTE OF THE DAY:
Never expect people to treat you any better than you treat yourself.
— Bo Bennett

HOW CAN I IMPROVE?

WHO CAN I ENCOURAGE OR PRAY FOR TODAY?

1.

MY COMMITMENT TO MYSELF TODAY:

2.

3.

LET IT ALL OUT!

WRITE YOUR FOOD STRUGGLES, MOTIVATION ISSUES, OR EVEN TRACK YOUR SUPPS AND MACROS.

DATE		DAY		TIME		WT	
MOOD				ENERGY LEVEL		1 2 3 4 5	
PROGRAM				PARTNER			

MUSCLE FOCUS			LOCATION					
STRENGTH TRAINING	S1	S2	S3	S4	S5	SET TYPE	EQUIP-MENT	P.R.

CALS BURNED	END TIME		DURATION	
CARDIO	DURATION	DISTANCE		INTENSITY

CALS BURNED	SUPPS USED	
HOW WAS MY WORKOUT?	1 2 3 4 5 6 7 8 9 10	

HYDRATE!

AIM TO CHECK OFF ALL 16 BOXES, ESPECIALLY ON WORKOUT DAYS.

| 1 | = 8 OZ |

2	3	4	5	6
7	8	9	10	11
12	13	14	15	16

FIT TIP:
Any increase in carb-o-HYDRATEs will result in temporary water weight gain. Understand this is to be expected with any increase in carbs.

WHAT AM I DOING WELL?

QUOTE OF THE DAY:
Well done is better than well said.
— Benjamin Franklin

HOW CAN I IMPROVE?

WHO CAN I ENCOURAGE OR PRAY FOR TODAY?

1.

MY COMMITMENT TO MYSELF TODAY:

2.

3.

LET IT ALL OUT!

WRITE YOUR FOOD STRUGGLES, MOTIVATION ISSUES, OR EVEN TRACK YOUR SUPPS AND MACROS.

DATE   DAY   TIME   WT
MOOD   ENERGY LEVEL   1 2 3 4 5
PROGRAM   PARTNER

MUSCLE FOCUS						LOCATION			
STRENGTH TRAINING	S1	S2	S3	S4	S5	SET TYPE	EQUIP-MENT	P.R.

CALS BURNED	END TIME		DURATION	
CARDIO	DURATION	DISTANCE		INTENSITY

CALS BURNED	SUPPS USED									
HOW WAS MY WORKOUT?	1	2	3	4	5	6	7	8	9	10

HYDRATE!

1 = 8 OZ

AIM TO CHECK OFF ALL 16 BOXES, ESPECIALLY ON WORKOUT DAYS.

2	3	4	5	6
7	8	9	10	11
12	13	14	15	16

FIT TIP:
When others don't support you, remember that your discipline and willpower just serves as uncomfortable reminder of what they lack.

WHAT AM I DOING WELL?

QUOTE OF THE DAY:
Everything comes to those who hustle while they wait.
— Thomas Edison

HOW CAN I IMPROVE?

WHO CAN I ENCOURAGE OR PRAY FOR TODAY?

1.

MY COMMITMENT TO MYSELF TODAY:

2.

3.

LET IT ALL OUT!

WRITE YOUR FOOD STRUGGLES, MOTIVATION ISSUES, OR EVEN TRACK YOUR SUPPS AND MACROS.

DATE		DAY		TIME		WT	
MOOD				ENERGY LEVEL		**1** 2 3 4 5	
PROGRAM				PARTNER			

MUSCLE FOCUS				LOCATION				
STRENGTH TRAINING	S1	S2	S3	S4	S5	SET TYPE	EQUIP- MENT	P.R.

CALS BURNED	END TIME		DURATION	
CARDIO	DURATION	DISTANCE		INTENSITY

CALS BURNED	SUPPS USED	
HOW WAS MY WORKOUT?	1 2 3 4 5 6 7 8 9 **10**	

HYDRATE!

☐ = 8 OZ

AIM TO CHECK OFF ALL 16 BOXES, ESPECIALLY ON WORKOUT DAYS.

1	2	3	4	5	6
7	8	9	10	11	
12	13	14	15	16	

FIT TIP:
Strength training will *not* make you bulky. It will change your body shape, improve your metabolism, and help you feel comfortable in your own skin.

WHAT AM I DOING WELL?

QUOTE OF THE DAY:
Dream as if you'll live forever...live as if you'll die today.
— James Dean

HOW CAN I IMPROVE?

WHO CAN I ENCOURAGE OR PRAY FOR TODAY?

1.

MY COMMITMENT TO MYSELF TODAY:

2.

3.

LET IT ALL OUT!

WRITE YOUR FOOD STRUGGLES, MOTIVATION ISSUES, OR EVEN TRACK YOUR SUPPS AND MACROS.

DATE		DAY		TIME		WT	
MOOD				ENERGY LEVEL		1 2 3 4 5	
PROGRAM				PARTNER			

MUSCLE FOCUS				LOCATION				
STRENGTH TRAINING	S1	S2	S3	S4	S5	SET TYPE	EQUIP-MENT	P.R.

CALS BURNED	END TIME		DURATION	
CARDIO	DURATION	DISTANCE		INTENSITY

CALS BURNED	SUPPS USED	
HOW WAS MY WORKOUT?		1 2 3 4 5 6 7 8 9 10

HYDRATE!

AIM TO CHECK OFF ALL 16 BOXES, ESPECIALLY ON WORKOUT DAYS.

1 = 8 OZ

1	2	3	4	5	6
7	8	9	10	11	
12	13	14	15	16	

FIT TIP:
If you know the scale will affect your mood or your decisions, avoid it.

WHAT AM I DOING WELL?

QUOTE OF THE DAY:
For God has not given us a spirit of fear and timidity, but of power, love and self-discipline.
— 2 Timothy 1:7

HOW CAN I IMPROVE?

WHO CAN I ENCOURAGE OR PRAY FOR TODAY?

1.

MY COMMITMENT TO MYSELF TODAY:

2.

3.

LET IT ALL OUT!

WRITE YOUR FOOD STRUGGLES, MOTIVATION ISSUES, OR EVEN TRACK YOUR SUPPS AND MACROS.

DATE		DAY		TIME		WT	
MOOD				ENERGY LEVEL		1 2 3 4 5	
PROGRAM				PARTNER			

MUSCLE FOCUS			LOCATION					
STRENGTH TRAINING	S1	S2	S3	S4	S5	SET TYPE	EQUIP-MENT	P.R.

CALS BURNED	END TIME		DURATION	
CARDIO	DURATION	DISTANCE		INTENSITY

CALS BURNED	SUPPS USED	
HOW WAS MY WORKOUT?		1 2 3 4 5 6 7 8 9 10

HYDRATE!

☐ = 8 OZ

AIM TO CHECK OFF ALL 16 BOXES, ESPECIALLY ON WORKOUT DAYS.

1	2	3	4	5	6
7	8	9	10	11
12	13	14	15	16

FIT TIP:

Question *everything*. Why you want to eat, what you hope to accomplish with your workouts, etc. You'll learn about yourself and will make better decisions.

WHAT AM I DOING WELL?

QUOTE OF THE DAY:

There are no traffic jams on the extra mile.

— Zig Ziglar

HOW CAN I IMPROVE?

WHO CAN I ENCOURAGE OR PRAY FOR TODAY?

1.

MY COMMITMENT TO MYSELF TODAY:

2.

3.

LET IT ALL OUT!

WRITE YOUR FOOD STRUGGLES, MOTIVATION ISSUES, OR EVEN TRACK YOUR SUPPS AND MACROS.

DATE		DAY		TIME		WT	

MOOD   ENERGY LEVEL   **1 2 3 4 5**

PROGRAM   PARTNER

MUSCLE FOCUS				LOCATION				
STRENGTH TRAINING	S1	S2	S3	S4	S5	SET TYPE	EQUIPMENT	P.R.

CALS BURNED	END TIME		DURATION	
CARDIO	DURATION	DISTANCE		INTENSITY

CALS BURNED	SUPPS USED									
HOW WAS MY WORKOUT?	1	2	3	4	5	6	7	8	9	10

HYDRATE!

AIM TO CHECK OFF ALL 16 BOXES, ESPECIALLY ON WORKOUT DAYS.

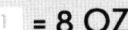 = 8 OZ

1	2	3	4	5	6
7	8	9	10	11
12	13	14	15	16

FIT TIP:
Keep healthy snacks handy at all times. Nothing will kill your progress faster than allowing yourself to get too hungry.

WHAT AM I DOING WELL?

QUOTE OF THE DAY:
The best way to predict the future is to create it.
— Peter Drucker

HOW CAN I IMPROVE?

WHO CAN I ENCOURAGE OR PRAY FOR TODAY?

1.

MY COMMITMENT TO MYSELF TODAY:

2.

3.

LET IT ALL OUT!

WRITE YOUR FOOD STRUGGLES, MOTIVATION ISSUES, OR EVEN TRACK YOUR SUPPS AND MACROS.

If you don't track your workout, it didn't happen!

Order another "My **GYM** Brain" today — never be without it!

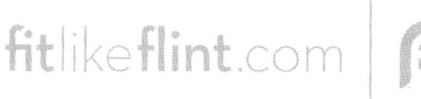

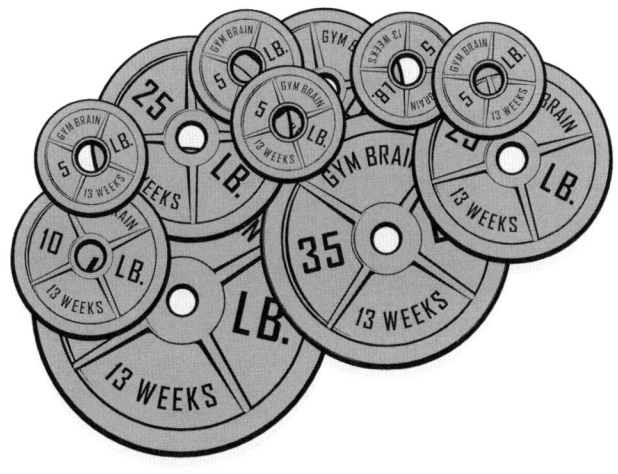

MY GYM BRAIN

A COMPREHENSIVE 13-WEEK FITNESS JOURNAL

fitlikeflint.com

IF YOU FAIL TO PLAN...

GOALS FOR THIS WEEK
Specific | **M**easurable | **A**ttainable | **R**ealistic | **T**ime-Bound

Example: I will drink one gallon of water each day this week.

1.

2.

3.

POTIENTIAL ROADBLOCKS

Anticipate what might throw you off track and plan a solution.

HAZARD: Business luncheon Thurs.

DETOUR: Protein shake before lunch

HAZARD:

DETOUR:

HAZARD:

DETOUR

VECTOR CHECK

Check each of your written goals and evaluate your progress.

Are you on track to meet your goal?

If not, why?

What can you do to get back on track?

If you need to modify your goals, do it now!

...YOU ARE PLANNING TO FAIL.
— Benjamin Franklin

MEAL PLANNING
Plan a menu - OR - Write down your meals - OR - Make a grocery list.

SUNDAY

MONDAY

TUESDAY

WEDNESDAY

THURSDAY

FRIDAY
Caution: weekend ahead!

SATURDAY

EXAMPLE A

M1 - oats, protein shake
M2 - whole grain toast & cheese
M3 - scrambled egg white sandwich w/spinach
M4 - carrots & hummus
M5 - chicken, rice, veggies
M6 - pizza (oops!)

EXAMPLE B

- Make turkey chili and protein bars

- Go grocery shopping

- Date Night! Look up restaurant menu

DATE		DAY		TIME		WT	

MOOD　　　　　　　ENERGY LEVEL　**1 2 3 4 5**

PROGRAM　　　　　　　PARTNER

MUSCLE FOCUS					LOCATION			
STRENGTH TRAINING	S1	S2	S3	S4	S5	SET TYPE	EQUIP-MENT	P.R.

CALS BURNED	END TIME		DURATION	
CARDIO	DURATION	DISTANCE		INTENSITY

CALS BURNED	SUPPS USED									
HOW WAS MY WORKOUT?	1	2	3	4	5	6	7	8	9	10

HYDRATE!

☐ = 8 OZ

AIM TO CHECK OFF ALL 16 BOXES, ESPECIALLY ON WORKOUT DAYS.

1	2	3	4	5	6
	7	8	9	10	11
	12	13	14	15	16

FIT TIP:
Know your triggers for making poor decisions. Emotions and hunger are just a few things that can cause you to derail. Have a plan.

WHAT AM I DOING WELL?

QUOTE OF THE DAY:
It is always too soon to quit!
— Norman Vincent Peale

HOW CAN I IMPROVE?

WHO CAN I ENCOURAGE OR PRAY FOR TODAY?

1.

MY COMMITMENT TO MYSELF TODAY:

2.

3.

LET IT ALL OUT!

WRITE YOUR FOOD STRUGGLES, MOTIVATION ISSUES, OR EVEN TRACK YOUR SUPPS AND MACROS.

DATE		DAY		TIME		WT	
MOOD				ENERGY LEVEL		1 2 3 4 5	
PROGRAM				PARTNER			

MUSCLE FOCUS				LOCATION				
STRENGTH TRAINING	S1	S2	S3	S4	S5	SET TYPE	EQUIPMENT	P.R.

CALS BURNED	END TIME		DURATION	
CARDIO	DURATION	DISTANCE		INTENSITY

CALS BURNED	SUPPS USED	
HOW WAS MY WORKOUT?	1 2 3 4 5 6 7 8 9 10	

HYDRATE!

AIM TO CHECK OFF ALL 16 BOXES, ESPECIALLY ON WORKOUT DAYS.

1 = 8 OZ

2	3	4	5	6
7	8	9	10	11
12	13	14	15	16

FIT TIP:
If it's not in your house, you can't eat it. Your children don't need it, either. So just don't keep it around.

WHAT AM I DOING WELL?

QUOTE OF THE DAY:
Expect the best. Prepare for the worst. Capitalize on what comes.
— Zig Ziglar

HOW CAN I IMPROVE?

WHO CAN I ENCOURAGE OR PRAY FOR TODAY?

1.

MY COMMITMENT TO MYSELF TODAY:

2.

3.

LET IT ALL OUT!

WRITE YOUR FOOD STRUGGLES, MOTIVATION ISSUES, OR EVEN TRACK YOUR SUPPS AND MACROS.

DATE		DAY		TIME		WT	
MOOD				ENERGY LEVEL		1 2 3 4 5	
PROGRAM				PARTNER			

MUSCLE FOCUS / LOCATION

STRENGTH TRAINING	S1	S2	S3	S4	S5	SET TYPE	EQUIP-MENT	P.R.

CALS BURNED	END TIME		DURATION	
CARDIO	DURATION	DISTANCE		INTENSITY

CALS BURNED	SUPPS USED	
HOW WAS MY WORKOUT?	1 2 3 4 5 6 7 8 9 10	

HYDRATE!

1 = 8 OZ

AIM TO CHECK OFF ALL 16 BOXES, ESPECIALLY ON WORKOUT DAYS.

2	3	4	5	6
7	8	9	10	11
12	13	14	15	16

FIT TIP:
It only takes two weeks to develop a new habit. If you start today, in one year you can have TWENTY-SIX new positive habits!

WHAT AM I DOING WELL?

QUOTE OF THE DAY:
The price of greatness is responsibilities.
- Sir Winston Churchill

HOW CAN I IMPROVE?

WHO CAN I ENCOURAGE OR PRAY FOR TODAY?

1.

MY COMMITMENT TO MYSELF TODAY:

2.

3.

LET IT ALL OUT!

WRITE YOUR FOOD STRUGGLES, MOTIVATION ISSUES, OR EVEN TRACK YOUR SUPPS AND MACROS.

DATE		DAY		TIME		WT	
MOOD				ENERGY LEVEL		1 2 3 4 5	
PROGRAM				PARTNER			

MUSCLE FOCUS				LOCATION				
STRENGTH TRAINING	S1	S2	S3	S4	S5	SET TYPE	EQUIP-MENT	P.R.

CALS BURNED	END TIME		DURATION	
CARDIO	DURATION	DISTANCE		INTENSITY

CALS BURNED	SUPPS USED	
HOW WAS MY WORKOUT?		1 2 3 4 5 6 7 8 9 10

HYDRATE!

☐ = 8 OZ

AIM TO CHECK OFF ALL 16 BOXES, ESPECIALLY ON WORKOUT DAYS.

1	2	3	4	5	6
7	8	9	10	11
12	13	14	15	16

FIT TIP:

You are stronger than you think, and are capable of much more than you realize. Challenge yourself and see what happens.

WHAT AM I DOING WELL?

QUOTE OF THE DAY:

Experience is not what happens to you; it's what you do with what happens to you.

— Aldous Huxley

HOW CAN I IMPROVE?

WHO CAN I ENCOURAGE OR PRAY FOR TODAY?

1.

MY COMMITMENT TO MYSELF TODAY:

2.

3.

LET IT ALL OUT!

WRITE YOUR FOOD STRUGGLES, MOTIVATION ISSUES, OR EVEN TRACK YOUR SUPPS AND MACROS.

DATE		DAY		TIME		WT	
MOOD				ENERGY LEVEL		1 2 3 4 5	
PROGRAM				PARTNER			

MUSCLE FOCUS				LOCATION				
STRENGTH TRAINING	S1	S2	S3	S4	S5	SET TYPE	EQUIPMENT	P.R.

CALS BURNED	END TIME		DURATION	
CARDIO	DURATION	DISTANCE		INTENSITY

CALS BURNED	SUPPS USED	
HOW WAS MY WORKOUT?		1 2 3 4 5 6 7 8 9 10

HYDRATE!

☐ = 8 OZ

AIM TO CHECK OFF ALL 16 BOXES, ESPECIALLY ON WORKOUT DAYS.

1	2	3	4	5	6
7	8	9	10	11
12	13	14	15	16

FIT TIP:
When you're truly hungry, pretty much any food will sound great. If only one specific food sounds good, it's likely a craving, not hunger.

WHAT AM I DOING WELL?

QUOTE OF THE DAY:
You must learn to translate wisdom and strong feelings into labor.
— Jim Rohn

HOW CAN I IMPROVE?

WHO CAN I ENCOURAGE OR PRAY FOR TODAY?

1.

MY COMMITMENT TO MYSELF TODAY:

2.

3.

LET IT ALL OUT!

WRITE YOUR FOOD STRUGGLES, MOTIVATION ISSUES, OR EVEN TRACK YOUR SUPPS AND MACROS.

DATE		DAY		TIME		WT	
MOOD			ENERGY LEVEL		**1** 2 3 4 5		
PROGRAM			PARTNER				

MUSCLE FOCUS			LOCATION					
STRENGTH TRAINING	S1	S2	S3	S4	S5	SET TYPE	EQUIPMENT	P.R.

CALS BURNED	END TIME		DURATION	
CARDIO	DURATION	DISTANCE		INTENSITY

CALS BURNED	SUPPS USED	
HOW WAS MY WORKOUT?	1 2 3 4 5 6 7 8 9 10	

HYDRATE!

AIM TO CHECK OFF ALL 16 BOXES, ESPECIALLY ON WORKOUT DAYS.

1 = 8 OZ

1	2	3	4	5	6
7	8	9	10	11
12	13	14	15	16

FIT TIP:
When you are crunched for time, try a Tabata or HIIT workout. You can get an intense workout in just 10-15 minutes.

WHAT AM I DOING WELL?

QUOTE OF THE DAY:
The will to win is important, but the will to prepare is vital.

— Joe Paterno

HOW CAN I IMPROVE?

WHO CAN I ENCOURAGE OR PRAY FOR TODAY?

1.

MY COMMITMENT TO MYSELF TODAY:

2.

3.

LET IT ALL OUT!

WRITE YOUR FOOD STRUGGLES, MOTIVATION ISSUES, OR EVEN TRACK YOUR SUPPS AND MACROS.

DATE		DAY		TIME		WT	
MOOD				ENERGY LEVEL		1 2 3 4 5	
PROGRAM				PARTNER			

MUSCLE FOCUS				LOCATION				
STRENGTH TRAINING	S1	S2	S3	S4	S5	SET TYPE	EQUIP-MENT	P.R.

CALS BURNED	END TIME		DURATION	
CARDIO	DURATION	DISTANCE		INTENSITY

CALS BURNED	SUPPS USED	
HOW WAS MY WORKOUT?		1 2 3 4 5 6 7 8 9 10

HYDRATE!

☐ = 8 OZ

AIM TO CHECK OFF ALL 16 BOXES, ESPECIALLY ON WORKOUT DAYS.

1	2	3	4	5	6
7	8	9	10	11
12	13	14	15	16

FIT TIP:
If your budget is limited (and whose isn't?), purchase some used fitness equipment. You can find nearly new equipment for half the cost of retail.

WHAT AM I DOING WELL?

QUOTE OF THE DAY:
Procrastination is opportunity's assassin.
— Victor Kiam

HOW CAN I IMPROVE?

WHO CAN I ENCOURAGE OR PRAY FOR TODAY?

1.

MY COMMITMENT TO MYSELF TODAY:

2.

3.

LET IT ALL OUT!

WRITE YOUR FOOD STRUGGLES, MOTIVATION ISSUES, OR EVEN TRACK YOUR SUPPS AND MACROS.

IF YOU FAIL TO PLAN...

GOALS FOR THIS WEEK
Specific | **M**easurable | **A**ttainable | **R**ealistic | **T**ime-Bound

Example: I will drink one gallon of water each day this week.

1.

2.

3.

POTIENTIAL ROADBLOCKS	VECTOR CHECK
Anticipate what might throw you off track and plan a solution.	Check each of your written goals and evaluate your progress.
HAZARD: Business luncheon Thurs.	Are you on track to meet your goal?
DETOUR: Protein shake before lunch	
HAZARD:	
	If not, why?
DETOUR:	
HAZARD:	What can you do to get back on track?
DETOUR	
	If you need to modify your goals, do it now!

...YOU ARE PLANNING TO FAIL.

— Benjamin Franklin

MEAL PLANNING
Plan a menu - OR - Write down your meals - OR - Make a grocery list.

SUNDAY

MONDAY

TUESDAY

WEDNESDAY

THURSDAY

FRIDAY
Caution: weekend ahead!

SATURDAY

EXAMPLE A

- M1 - oats, protein shake
- M2 - whole grain toast & cheese
- M3 - scrambled egg white sandwich w/spinach
- M4 - carrots & hummus
- M5 - chicken, rice, veggies
- M6 - pizza (oops!)

EXAMPLE B

- Make turkey chili and protein bars
- Go grocery shopping
- Date Night! Look up restaurant menu

DATE		DAY		TIME		WT	
MOOD				ENERGY LEVEL		1 2 3 4 5	
PROGRAM				PARTNER			

MUSCLE FOCUS				LOCATION				
STRENGTH TRAINING	S1	S2	S3	S4	S5	SET TYPE	EQUIPMENT	P.R.

CALS BURNED	END TIME		DURATION	
CARDIO	DURATION	DISTANCE		INTENSITY

CALS BURNED	SUPPS USED	
HOW WAS MY WORKOUT?	1 2 3 4 5 6 7 8 9 10	

HYDRATE!

AIM TO CHECK OFF ALL 16 BOXES, ESPECIALLY ON WORKOUT DAYS.

1	= 8 OZ			
2	3	4	5	6
7	8	9	10	11
12	13	14	15	16

FIT TIP:
Start a blog or social media account to chronicle your fitness journey. You will be surprised at how many people are eager to cheer you on!

WHAT AM I DOING WELL?

QUOTE OF THE DAY:
Great things are not done by impulse, but by a series of small things brought together.
— Vincent Van Gogh

HOW CAN I IMPROVE?

WHO CAN I ENCOURAGE OR PRAY FOR TODAY?

1.

MY COMMITMENT TO MYSELF TODAY:

2.

3.

LET IT ALL OUT!

WRITE YOUR FOOD STRUGGLES, MOTIVATION ISSUES, OR EVEN TRACK YOUR SUPPS AND MACROS.

DATE		DAY		TIME		WT	
MOOD				ENERGY LEVEL		1 2 3 4 5	
PROGRAM				PARTNER			

MUSCLE FOCUS				LOCATION			
STRENGTH TRAINING	S1	S2	S3	S4	S5	SET TYPE	EQUIPMENT	P.R.

CALS BURNED	END TIME		DURATION	
CARDIO	DURATION	DISTANCE		INTENSITY

CALS BURNED	SUPPS USED	
HOW WAS MY WORKOUT?	1 2 3 4 5 6 7 8 9 10	

HYDRATE!

1 = 8 OZ

AIM TO CHECK OFF ALL 16 BOXES, ESPECIALLY ON WORKOUT DAYS.

1	2	3	4	5	6
7	8	9	10	11
12	13	14	15	16

FIT TIP:
When you reach a fitness goal, avoid food rewards. Instead, reward yourself with a manicure, blowout, or new gym gear!

WHAT AM I DOING WELL?

QUOTE OF THE DAY:
All our dreams can come true - if we have the courage to pursue them.
— Walt Disney

HOW CAN I IMPROVE?

WHO CAN I ENCOURAGE OR PRAY FOR TODAY?

1.

MY COMMITMENT TO MYSELF TODAY:

2.

3.

LET IT ALL OUT!

WRITE YOUR FOOD STRUGGLES, MOTIVATION ISSUES, OR EVEN TRACK YOUR SUPPS AND MACROS.

DATE		DAY		TIME		WT	
MOOD				ENERGY LEVEL		1 2 3 4 5	
PROGRAM				PARTNER			

MUSCLE FOCUS				LOCATION				
STRENGTH TRAINING	S1	S2	S3	S4	S5	SET TYPE	EQUIP-MENT	P.R.

CALS BURNED	END TIME		DURATION	
CARDIO	DURATION	DISTANCE		INTENSITY

CALS BURNED	SUPPS USED	
HOW WAS MY WORKOUT?	1 2 3 4 5 6 7 8 9 10	

HYDRATE!

☐ = 8 OZ

AIM TO CHECK OFF ALL 16 BOXES, ESPECIALLY ON WORKOUT DAYS.

1	2	3	4	5	6
7	8	9	10	11
12	13	14	15	16

FIT TIP:
Smile at the new faces in your gym. Everyone can benefit from a kind word and a smile.

WHAT AM I DOING WELL?

QUOTE OF THE DAY:
You will never change your life until you change something you do daily. The secret of your success is found in your daily routine. — John Maxwell

HOW CAN I IMPROVE?

WHO CAN I ENCOURAGE OR PRAY FOR TODAY?

1.

MY COMMITMENT TO MYSELF TODAY:

2.

3.

LET IT ALL OUT!

WRITE YOUR FOOD STRUGGLES, MOTIVATION ISSUES, OR EVEN TRACK YOUR SUPPS AND MACROS.

DATE		DAY		TIME		WT		
MOOD				ENERGY LEVEL		1 2 3 4 5		
PROGRAM				PARTNER				

MUSCLE FOCUS			LOCATION					
STRENGTH TRAINING	S1	S2	S3	S4	S5	SET TYPE	EQUIPMENT	P.R.

CALS BURNED	END TIME		DURATION	
CARDIO	DURATION	DISTANCE		INTENSITY

CALS BURNED	SUPPS USED	
HOW WAS MY WORKOUT?		1 2 3 4 5 6 7 8 9 10

HYDRATE!

AIM TO CHECK OFF ALL 16 BOXES, ESPECIALLY ON WORKOUT DAYS.

1	= 8 OZ			
2	3	4	5	6
7	8	9	10	11
12	13	14	15	16

FIT TIP:
Drink 16-20 ounces of warm water first thing in the morning. Add a splash of lemon juice for improved digestion throughout the day.

WHAT AM I DOING WELL?

QUOTE OF THE DAY:
Once you say you're going to settle for second, that's what happens to you in life, I find.
— John F. Kennedy

HOW CAN I IMPROVE?

WHO CAN I ENCOURAGE OR PRAY FOR TODAY?

1.

MY COMMITMENT TO MYSELF TODAY:

2.

3.

LET IT ALL OUT!

WRITE YOUR FOOD STRUGGLES, MOTIVATION ISSUES, OR EVEN TRACK YOUR SUPPS AND MACROS.

DATE		DAY		TIME		WT	
MOOD				ENERGY LEVEL		**1** **2** **3** **4** **5**	
PROGRAM				PARTNER			

MUSCLE FOCUS				LOCATION					
STRENGTH TRAINING	S1	S2	S3	S4	S5	SET TYPE	EQUIP-MENT	P.R.

CALS BURNED	END TIME		DURATION	
CARDIO	DURATION	DISTANCE		INTENSITY

CALS BURNED	SUPPS USED	
HOW WAS MY WORKOUT?	**1** **2** **3** **4** **5** **6** **7** **8** **9** **10**	

HYDRATE!

AIM TO CHECK OFF ALL 16 BOXES, ESPECIALLY ON WORKOUT DAYS.

1	= 8 OZ

2	3	4	5	6
7	8	9	10	11
12	13	14	15	16

FIT TIP:
Ask for a "to go" container when you eat out, and immediately put half of your food in the box when your meal arrives. It's a great calorie *and* money saver.

WHAT AM I DOING WELL?

QUOTE OF THE DAY:
Finish each day and be done with it. You have done what you could.
— Ralph Waldo Emerson

HOW CAN I IMPROVE?

WHO CAN I ENCOURAGE OR PRAY FOR TODAY?

1.

MY COMMITMENT TO MYSELF TODAY:

2.

3.

LET IT ALL OUT!

WRITE YOUR FOOD STRUGGLES, MOTIVATION ISSUES, OR EVEN TRACK YOUR SUPPS AND MACROS.

DATE		DAY		TIME		WT	
MOOD				ENERGY LEVEL		1 2 3 4 5	
PROGRAM				PARTNER			

MUSCLE FOCUS				LOCATION				
STRENGTH TRAINING	S1	S2	S3	S4	S5	SET TYPE	EQUIPMENT	P.R.

CALS BURNED	END TIME		DURATION	
CARDIO	DURATION	DISTANCE		INTENSITY

CALS BURNED	SUPPS USED	
HOW WAS MY WORKOUT?		1 2 3 4 5 6 7 8 9 10

HYDRATE!

☐ = 8 OZ

AIM TO CHECK OFF ALL 16 BOXES, ESPECIALLY ON WORKOUT DAYS.

1	2	3	4	5	6
	7	8	9	10	11
	12	13	14	15	16

FIT TIP:
Instead of focusing on the foods you *can't* have, focus instead on the foods you *want* to nourish your body.

WHAT AM I DOING WELL?

QUOTE OF THE DAY:
Work harder on yourself than you do on your job.
— Jim Rohn

HOW CAN I IMPROVE?

WHO CAN I ENCOURAGE OR PRAY FOR TODAY?

1.

MY COMMITMENT TO MYSELF TODAY:

2.

3.

LET IT ALL OUT!

WRITE YOUR FOOD STRUGGLES, MOTIVATION ISSUES, OR EVEN TRACK YOUR SUPPS AND MACROS.

DATE　　　　　　DAY　　　　　　TIME　　　　　　WT
MOOD　　　　　　　　　ENERGY LEVEL　　1　2　3　4　5
PROGRAM　　　　　　　　　　PARTNER

MUSCLE FOCUS			LOCATION					
STRENGTH TRAINING	S1	S2	S3	S4	S5	SET TYPE	EQUIP-MENT	P.R.

CALS BURNED	END TIME		DURATION	
CARDIO	DURATION	DISTANCE		INTENSITY

CALS BURNED	SUPPS USED	
HOW WAS MY WORKOUT?	1　2　3　4　5　6　7　8　9　10	

HYDRATE!

AIM TO CHECK OFF ALL 16 BOXES, ESPECIALLY ON WORKOUT DAYS.

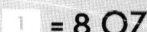 = 8 OZ

1	2	3	4	5	6
7	8	9	10	11
12	13	14	15	16

FIT TIP:
Try something new to mix things up. Incorporate a stretching routine, yoga, kickboxing, or some other new aspect into your training.

WHAT AM I DOING WELL?

QUOTE OF THE DAY:
Visualization is daydreaming with a purpose.
— Bo Bennett

HOW CAN I IMPROVE?

WHO CAN I ENCOURAGE OR PRAY FOR TODAY?

1.

MY COMMITMENT TO MYSELF TODAY:

2.

3.

LET IT ALL OUT!

WRITE YOUR FOOD STRUGGLES, MOTIVATION ISSUES, OR EVEN TRACK YOUR SUPPS AND MACROS.

IF YOU FAIL TO PLAN...

GOALS FOR THIS WEEK
Specific | **M**easurable | **A**ttainable | **R**ealistic | **T**ime-Bound

Example: I will drink one gallon of water each day this week.

1.

2.

3.

POTIENTIAL ROADBLOCKS	VECTOR CHECK
Anticipate what might throw you off track and plan a solution.	Check each of your written goals and evaluate your progress.
HAZARD: Business luncheon Thurs.	Are you on track to meet your goal?
DETOUR: Protein shake before lunch	
HAZARD:	
	If not, why?
DETOUR:	
HAZARD:	What can you do to get back on track?
DETOUR	
	If you need to modify your goals, do it now!

...YOU ARE PLANNING TO FAIL.

— Benjamin Franklin

MEAL PLANNING
Plan a menu - OR - Write down your meals - OR - Make a grocery list.

SUNDAY

MONDAY

TUESDAY

WEDNESDAY

THURSDAY

FRIDAY
Caution: weekend ahead!

SATURDAY

EXAMPLE A

M1 - oats, protein shake
M2 - whole grain toast & cheese
M3 - scrambled egg white sandwich w/spinach
M4 - carrots & hummus
M5 - chicken, rice, veggies
M6 - pizza (oops!)

EXAMPLE B

- Make turkey chili and protein bars

- Go grocery shopping

- Date Night! Look up restaurant menu

DATE   DAY   TIME   WT
MOOD   ENERGY LEVEL   **1 2 3 4 5**
PROGRAM   PARTNER

MUSCLE FOCUS			LOCATION				
STRENGTH TRAINING	S1	S2	S3	S4	S5	SET TYPE	EQUIP-MENT	P.R.

CALS BURNED	END TIME		DURATION	
CARDIO	DURATION	DISTANCE		INTENSITY

CALS BURNED	SUPPS USED	
HOW WAS MY WORKOUT?	**1 2 3 4 5 6 7 8 9 10**	

HYDRATE!

1 = 8 OZ

AIM TO CHECK OFF ALL 16 BOXES, ESPECIALLY ON WORKOUT DAYS.

2	3	4	5	6
7	8	9	10	11
12	13	14	15	16

FIT TIP:
Find a workout partner. Even loners can benefit from occasional workouts with a partner.

WHAT AM I DOING WELL?

QUOTE OF THE DAY:
Our lives are a sum total of the choices we have made.
                                    - Wayne Dyer

HOW CAN I IMPROVE?

WHO CAN I ENCOURAGE OR PRAY FOR TODAY?

1.

MY COMMITMENT TO MYSELF TODAY:

2.

3.

LET IT ALL OUT!

WRITE YOUR FOOD STRUGGLES, MOTIVATION ISSUES, OR EVEN TRACK YOUR SUPPS AND MACROS.

DATE _____ DAY _____ TIME _____ WT _____
MOOD _____ ENERGY LEVEL 1 2 3 4 5
PROGRAM _____ PARTNER _____

MUSCLE FOCUS			LOCATION					
STRENGTH TRAINING	S1	S2	S3	S4	S5	SET TYPE	EQUIP-MENT	P.R.

CALS BURNED	END TIME		DURATION	
CARDIO	DURATION	DISTANCE		INTENSITY

CALS BURNED	SUPPS USED									
HOW WAS MY WORKOUT?	1	2	3	4	5	6	7	8	9	10

HYDRATE!

AIM TO CHECK OFF ALL 16 BOXES, ESPECIALLY ON WORKOUT DAYS.

1 = 8 OZ

1	2	3	4	5	6
7	8	9	10	11
12	13	14	15	16

FIT TIP:
For maximum fat burning benefits, do cardio immediately after a lifting session.

WHAT AM I DOING WELL?

QUOTE OF THE DAY:
Perpetual optimism is a force multiplier.
— Colin Powell

HOW CAN I IMPROVE?

WHO CAN I ENCOURAGE OR PRAY FOR TODAY?

1.

MY COMMITMENT TO MYSELF TODAY:

2.

3.

LET IT ALL OUT!

WRITE YOUR FOOD STRUGGLES, MOTIVATION ISSUES, OR EVEN TRACK YOUR SUPPS AND MACROS.

DATE　　　　　　　DAY　　　　　　TIME　　　　　　WT
MOOD　　　　　　　　　　　ENERGY LEVEL　**1** 2 3 4 5
PROGRAM　　　　　　　　　　　　PARTNER

MUSCLE FOCUS						LOCATION		
STRENGTH TRAINING	S1	S2	S3	S4	S5	SET TYPE	EQUIP-MENT	P.R.

CALS BURNED	END TIME		DURATION	
CARDIO	DURATION	DISTANCE		INTENSITY

CALS BURNED	SUPPS USED									
HOW WAS MY WORKOUT?	1	2	3	4	5	6	7	8	9	10

HYDRATE!

1 = 8 OZ

AIM TO CHECK OFF ALL 16 BOXES, ESPECIALLY ON WORKOUT DAYS.

1	2	3	4	5	6
	7	8	9	10	11
	12	13	14	15	16

FIT TIP:
When you don't want to exercise, commit to ten minutes. You'll likely feel energized and ready to finish. If you still feel awful, quit and rest.

WHAT AM I DOING WELL?

QUOTE OF THE DAY:
So simple, but true...Nothing will work unless you do.
— Maya Angelou

HOW CAN I IMPROVE?

WHO CAN I ENCOURAGE OR PRAY FOR TODAY?

1.

MY COMMITMENT TO MYSELF TODAY:

2.

3.

LET IT ALL OUT!

WRITE YOUR FOOD STRUGGLES, MOTIVATION ISSUES, OR EVEN TRACK YOUR SUPPS AND MACROS.

DATE		DAY		TIME		WT	
MOOD				ENERGY LEVEL		1 2 3 4 5	
PROGRAM				PARTNER			

MUSCLE FOCUS				LOCATION				
STRENGTH TRAINING	S1	S2	S3	S4	S5	SET TYPE	EQUIP-MENT	P.R.

CALS BURNED	END TIME		DURATION	
CARDIO	DURATION	DISTANCE		INTENSITY

CALS BURNED	SUPPS USED	
HOW WAS MY WORKOUT?	1 2 3 4 5 6 7 8 9 10	

HYDRATE!

AIM TO CHECK OFF ALL 16 BOXES, ESPECIALLY ON WORKOUT DAYS.

| 1 | = 8 OZ |

2	3	4	5	6
7	8	9	10	11
12	13	14	15	16

FIT TIP:
If it doesn't help you reach your goals, it's keeping you from them.

WHAT AM I DOING WELL?

QUOTE OF THE DAY:
There are two major pains in life. One is the pain of discipline, the other is the pain of regret.
— Jim Rohn

HOW CAN I IMPROVE?

WHO CAN I ENCOURAGE OR PRAY FOR TODAY?

1.

MY COMMITMENT TO MYSELF TODAY:

2.

3.

LET IT ALL OUT!

WRITE YOUR FOOD STRUGGLES, MOTIVATION ISSUES, OR EVEN TRACK YOUR SUPPS AND MACROS.

DATE		DAY		TIME		WT	
MOOD				ENERGY LEVEL		1 2 3 4 5	
PROGRAM				PARTNER			

MUSCLE FOCUS				LOCATION				
STRENGTH TRAINING	S1	S2	S3	S4	S5	SET TYPE	EQUIP-MENT	P.R.

CALS BURNED	END TIME		DURATION	
CARDIO	DURATION	DISTANCE		INTENSITY

CALS BURNED	SUPPS USED	
HOW WAS MY WORKOUT?	1 2 3 4 5 6 7 8 9 10	

HYDRATE!

AIM TO CHECK OFF ALL 16 BOXES, ESPECIALLY ON WORKOUT DAYS.

1	= 8 OZ			
2	3	4	5	6
7	8	9	10	11
12	13	14	15	16

FIT TIP:
Bring a healthy snack to the grocery store. *Never* go when you are hungry or poor decisions will likely be rampant.

WHAT AM I DOING WELL?

QUOTE OF THE DAY:
Without a struggle, there can be no progress.
— Frederick Douglass

HOW CAN I IMPROVE?

WHO CAN I ENCOURAGE OR PRAY FOR TODAY?

1.

MY COMMITMENT TO MYSELF TODAY:

2.

3.

LET IT ALL OUT!

WRITE YOUR FOOD STRUGGLES, MOTIVATION ISSUES, OR EVEN TRACK YOUR SUPPS AND MACROS.

DATE _____ DAY _____ TIME _____ WT _____
MOOD _____ ENERGY LEVEL 1 2 3 4 5
PROGRAM _____ PARTNER _____

MUSCLE FOCUS					LOCATION			
STRENGTH TRAINING	S1	S2	S3	S4	S5	SET TYPE	EQUIP-MENT	P.R.

CALS BURNED	END TIME		DURATION	
CARDIO	DURATION	DISTANCE		INTENSITY

CALS BURNED	SUPPS USED									
HOW WAS MY WORKOUT?	1	2	3	4	5	6	7	8	9	10

HYDRATE!

AIM TO CHECK OFF ALL 16 BOXES, ESPECIALLY ON WORKOUT DAYS.

[1] = 8 OZ

1	2	3	4	5	6
7	8	9	10	11
12	13	14	15	16

FIT TIP:
It's wise to slowly increase your calories to maintenance for a short period of time every 12-16 weeks to help reset your metabolism.

WHAT AM I DOING WELL?

QUOTE OF THE DAY:
Great spirits have always encountered violent opposition from mediocre minds.
— Albert Einstein

HOW CAN I IMPROVE?

WHO CAN I ENCOURAGE OR PRAY FOR TODAY?

1.

MY COMMITMENT TO MYSELF TODAY:

2.

3.

LET IT ALL OUT!

WRITE YOUR FOOD STRUGGLES, MOTIVATION ISSUES, OR EVEN TRACK YOUR SUPPS AND MACROS.

DATE		DAY		TIME		WT	
MOOD				ENERGY LEVEL		1 2 3 4 5	
PROGRAM				PARTNER			

MUSCLE FOCUS				LOCATION				
STRENGTH TRAINING	S1	S2	S3	S4	S5	SET TYPE	EQUIPMENT	P.R.

CALS BURNED	END TIME		DURATION	
CARDIO	DURATION	DISTANCE		INTENSITY

CALS BURNED	SUPPS USED	
HOW WAS MY WORKOUT?		1 2 3 4 5 6 7 8 9 10

HYDRATE!

AIM TO CHECK OFF ALL 16 BOXES, ESPECIALLY ON WORKOUT DAYS.

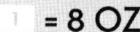 = 8 OZ

1	2	3	4	5	6
7	8	9	10	11	
12	13	14	15	16	

FIT TIP:
If you find yourself struggling with nutrition, temporarily allow yourself more calories to prevent a binge. Drop calories back down when recovered.

WHAT AM I DOING WELL?

QUOTE OF THE DAY:
The best way out is always through.
— Robert Frost

HOW CAN I IMPROVE?

WHO CAN I ENCOURAGE OR PRAY FOR TODAY?

1.

MY COMMITMENT TO MYSELF TODAY:

2.

3.

LET IT ALL OUT!

WRITE YOUR FOOD STRUGGLES, MOTIVATION ISSUES, OR EVEN TRACK YOUR SUPPS AND MACROS.

CONNECT WITH ME!

- @fitlikeflint
- @fitlikeflint
- Fit Like Flint

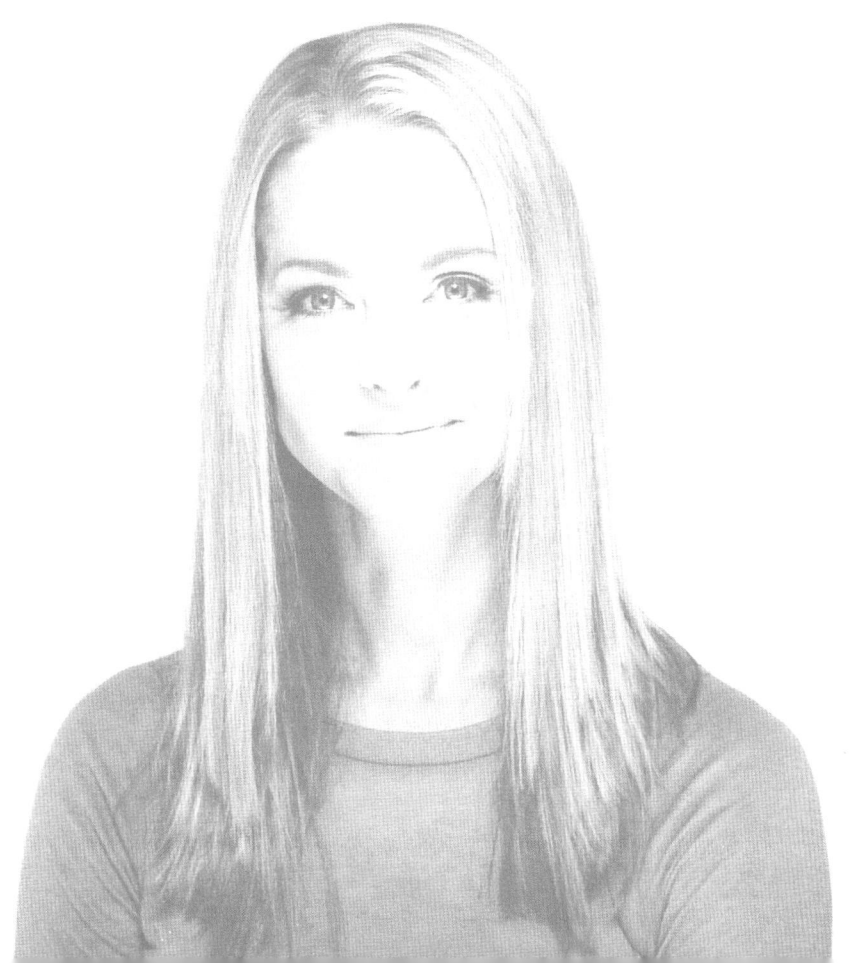

WITH A THANKFUL HEART:

Goal chasing can be a lonely, misunderstood business. The Lord has blessed me with people who support and encourage me, and speak the truth when I need to hear it. I am humbled and blessed to call them my family and friends.

To my very *best* friend, my husband, Ben: I never knew our lives would be such a roller coaster! Spending my life with you has been more exhilarating (and sometimes more terrifying!) than I ever imagined. Our life is a roller coaster, to put it mildly, but I wouldn't want to go through life's highs and lows with anyone but you. Without your love and your support, I never would have made it this far. Thank you for being a listening ear on all my "give up days" and encouraging me to keep going.

To my children, Katie, Maggie, and Colin: Thank you for being so supportive and patient as I worked on this project. I know hearing "Just a minute," "When I get done with this section," or "Maybe later" was difficult, but you handled it like champs. I love you so much. Now, let's head to the playground!

To my parents: Thank you for your love and support. Dad, thank you for sharing your marketing knowledge and business experience with me over the past few years. I had no idea I'd gained your entrepreneurial spirit! If I had known you were so knowledgeable, maybe I would've listened a little better during my teenage years. (Nah, probably not.) Mom, thank you for being a sounding board and a listening ear for all my ideas. Thanks to both of you for being so willing to watch our children while we were paying our dues at countless bodybuilding shows and fitness expos.

To my parents-in-law: Thank you for raising an incredible son who is now a phenomenal husband. Thank you for your support as we've ventured off the beaten path. I will never forget you spending so much of your vacation time helping us ship our very first FLF apparel nearly three years ago. I was humbled and grateful then, and remain so to this day.

To Clint Walkingstick: Thank you for providing incredible design, business mentorship, and friendship over the past three years. You make us look good… no…GREAT, and we're very thankful for all you do. You're one of a kind, and I really don't think you look stupid at all! :-) (If you have a business, hire WalkingstickDesign.com to make it look polished and professional.)

To the women of Relentless 2.0: You ladies are the reason I do what I do. You trusted me in the beginning, and our fitness group has been such incredible motivation and accountability for me. Thank you for all your input on this project. I can't wait to see what all of us accomplish in the future by supporting and encouraging each other! I'm so proud of you and blessed to have the absolute *best* virtual friends!

To Jamie (Eason) Middleton: Once my fitspiration, and now my friend (and *still* my fitspiration). You are a shining light in the fitness industry. I'm so thankful for you and Michael and the example you set for others. I admire the woman you are and the woman you're working to become.

To Laura Grubb: Thank you for creating the Brainiacs characters and for adding several Fit Tips to this fitness journal. Your feedback and input was invaluable and I'm so thankful for all your help on this project.

To Carrie Wilkerson: My dad recommended long ago that I read your book <u>The Barefoot Executive</u>, and I wish I'd done it right away instead of waiting *more than a year!* I love your passion for helping others, your candor, and your ambition. Thank you for setting a great example of a female entrepreneur who succeeds without sacrificing what matters most.

A few more who deserve to be thanked by name: These ladies in particular have listened to all my ideas and helped me sift through to decide which ones are worth keeping. They have flown across the country (or from out-of-country!) to fitness expos and business meetings on their own dime to help us simply because they believe in what we're doing.

When I was overwhelmed with the rapid growth of Fit Like Flint, they even stepped up to help me run the business. They are remarkable women that I am so blessed to call my friends.

Tannis Gregory
Colleen Howe
Tracey LaValle
Tiffany Riley
Mandy Mae Allen
Cari Clift
Melanie Gaines
Nicole Boyce
Kelley Smith
Amanda Thomas
Brooke Cowden

Most of all, I want to thank my Creator and Savior. As someone who was convinced I was devoid of all creativity, my husband reminded me that I was *created by the Creator to be creative*. God has given me a drive and passion that I never knew was in me. He has guided my decisions and given me countless opportunities to serve Him by serving others, and I'm so thankful for that.